STEPHEN HARROD BUHNER

❧

Sacred Plant Medicine:
Explorations in the Practice of Indigenous Herbalism

❧

One Spirit Many Peoples:
A Manifesto For Earth Spirituality

❧

Sacred and Herbal Healing Beers:
The Secrets of Ancient Fermentation

❧

Herbal Antibiotics:
Natural Alternatives for Drug-resistant Bacteria

❧

Herbs for Hepatitis C and the Liver

❧

The Lost Language of Plants:
The Ecological Importance of Plant Medicines to Life on Earth

❧

Vital Man: Natural Healthcare for Men at Midlife

❧

The Fasting Path:
The Way to Physical, Emotional, and Spiritual Healing and Renewal

❧

The Taste of Wild Water:
Poems and Stories Found While Walking in Woods

❧

The Secret Teachings of Plants:
The Intelligence of the Heart in the Direct Perception of Nature

Healing Lyme

Natural Prevention
and Treatment of
Lyme Borreliosis
and Its Coinfections

STEPHEN HARROD BUHNER

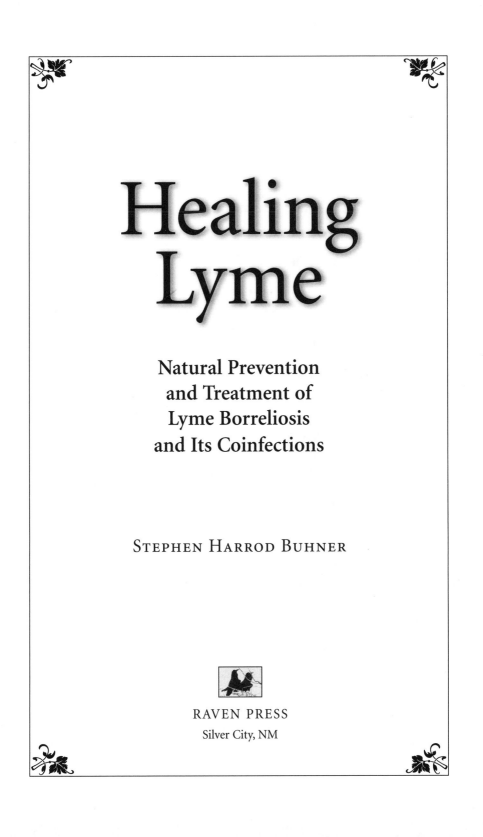

RAVEN PRESS

Silver City, NM

Raven Press
8 Pioneer Road
Silver City, NM 88061

This book is for educational purposes only. It is not intended to replace a qualified health care practitioner.

Publisher's Cataloging-in-Publication Data
Buhner, Stephen Harrod
    Healing lyme: natural healing and prevention for Lyme borreliosis and its coinfections/ Stephen Harrod Buhner.—1st ed.—Randolph, Vt.: Raven Press, 2005
        p. ; cm.
        Includes bibliographical references and index.
        ISBN10: 0-9708696-3-0
        ISBN13: 978-0-9708696-3-0
        1. Lyme disease. 2. Lyme disease—Alternative treatment.
    3. Herbs—Therapeutic use. I. Title.
    RC155.5 .B84 2005
    616.9/246—dc22   CIP

Printed and bound in the United States of America by Sheridan Books
10 9 8 7 6 5 4

INTERIOR DESIGN AND LAYOUT: Boulder Bookworks
TECHNICAL EDITOR: Paul Bergner

For those people

whose doctors told them

it was all in their heads

ACKNOWLEDGMENTS

All the people who asked me for this book for the past ten years: Wendy Leffel, who insisted; Fran Giaquinto for her research and help in London; Paul Bergner, who kept me honest; Mary Lou Quinn-Beatie of NAPRALERT, at the University of Chicago School of Pharmacy, who worked to get me the data I needed before they closed her down for lack of funding; the microbiologists who have no political agenda other than the truth; the physicians on the front lines; the *Borrelia* spirochetes, who taught me more than I ever wanted to know about cleverness; and the plants without whose lives none of us would be here.

CONTENTS

FOREWORD

by Wendy Leffel, M.D.

My own education about Lyme began shortly after I opened a private, holistic, consulting practice. Due to the nature of my practice many of my patients suffered from chronic illnesses that had not responded to mainstream, western medicine. A significant number of those were later found to have Lyme disease. I witnessed previously vital and intelligent people become increasingly debilitated. Time and again, I heard similar tragic stories by people who had been told by their health care providers that their numerous disabling symptoms were all in their heads. Because I had designed my practice to allow time to listen to people, I encouraged them to tell their stories. Through this more personal approach, I was able to see that their multiple, often confusing complaints, were not "just in their heads." These people were truly and terribly ill and searching desperately for a way to regain their health. I wondered why physicians weren't being given the information they needed to be able to recognize, diagnose, and treat this emerging disease.

I was fortunate, early on, to have a patient who had been battling Lyme disease for years and who was willing to share what she knew with me. Once pointed in the right direction, I began to search for clear, reliable information on Lyme. I was shocked at how difficult it was to come by, how little information was readily available on such a quickly-spreading, serious illness. Different sources on Lyme disease were often contradictory. I was repeatedly frustrated in my attempts to learn enough about Lyme to confidently treat the people who were suffering with it. I was appalled by the paucity of useful information available to physicians concerning Lyme disease and its coinfections. Even vital information on appropriate diagnostic tests was not available from mainstream sources. I realized that discerning fact from fiction would require months of intense, dedicated research. As a busy physician, I simply did not have the time to spend on such a search. And, people were suffering.

Many people who are infected with Lyme recover only partially, or temporarily, using appropriately prescribed antibiotics alone. In addition, Herxheimer (die-off) reactions resulting from successful antibiotic use can be severe. Clearly, another approach is needed.

This is the book I wish I had had when I was struggling to understand and treat Lyme disease. I am profoundly grateful to Stephen Buhner for accepting the daunting challenge of creating a well-researched, thorough, and comprehensive book. His detailed description of the mechanisms Lyme spirochetes use to invade the body, avoid detection, and cause physical damage will clarify this disease for people with Lyme, their families, and healing practitioners. The detailed information in this book fills a significant void.

Stephen's diligent work and deep understanding of this emerging disease has allowed him to craft an extremely elegant, much needed, herbal response. An herbal protocol, such as this one, that is capable of improving the efficacy of antibiotic treatment while relieving distressing symptoms, offers renewed hope to countless people. I am delighted by the exactness with which the herbs described in this book fit the physiological changes that occur in Lyme disease. The specificity with which this herbal protocol counters the mechanisms and deleterious effects of Lyme borrelia and its coinfections is extraordinary. The protocols contained in this book offer new opportunities for all those longing to reclaim their lives from this devastating disease.

As someone who lives in an area in which Lyme is rapidly becoming endemic, I am very relieved to read about preventive measures against Lyme borrelia. Lyme disease is spreading and will continue to spread, partly as a result of global warming. Taking extreme measures to exterminate current tick vectors (such as deer or mice), will result in the needless deaths of thousands of ecologically vital animals and simply cause ticks to change to new host animals. By taking a few herbs daily we can reduce our risk of developing Lyme while simultaneously supporting our overall health. To my mind, the benefits are well worth the small effort required.

In order to reduce the incidence of this disease, the education of health care professionals, the public and politicians about Lyme, needs to be addressed. This is the first book that makes reliable, scientifically-based information on Lyme readily accessible to everyone. While a few courageous, Lyme-literate practitioners exist, there are too few to address the needs of the increasing numbers of people who are being infected. I hope the valuable information in this book will enable more practitioners to recognize, diagnose, and successfully treat Lyme disease. We desperately need practitioners on the front lines who recognize and treat Lyme properly in the early, most curable stages and who take appropriately aggressive measures in later stages. I applaud all those who have been touched by Lyme borrelia and who have worked diligently to increase public and practitioner awareness of Lyme disease. Your mission is not an easy one. I hope this book will help.

A NOTE TO THE READER

This book is intended for people with Lyme disease, as well as practitioners who want to better understand the mechanics of the disease process and the Lyme borrelia organisms themselves. As a result, some parts of the book are more technical than others. If you are not reading this book for technical understanding, just skip the technical parts. There are boxed sections in each chapter outlining all the necessary herbs, supplements, and dosages for treating the disease.

Welcome to the Lyme Wars

W hen I began working on this book, I did not expect that I would be entering a war zone. It is not, however, a zone of conflict between human beings and Lyme disease organisms but a battle between people holding competing theories of Lyme disease and its treatment. The intensity of the conflict has regrettably reached almost religious levels amongst the different proponents. Caught in the cross-fire are those with Lyme disease who are trying to understand what is happening to them and to discover how best to deal with it. This is, in my opinion, reprehensible.

This is not a book that can resolve the Lyme wars. It was never my intention to take on such a complicated and overwhelming task. Other people, more capable than I, must do this; it is my hope they do so soon.

This book is, instead, a response to the many people who have asked me over the years for something to help them with Lyme disease and its symptoms. Regrettably, there is no way I can avoid the Lyme wars in the writing of this book, nor can you if you look very deeply into the matter yourself. So, the best I can do is to tell you that the conflict exists and that you will hear a lot of things about Lyme disease that will conflict with other information you find. Little of it will seem to make sense if you spend any time at all with the subject. (You may begin to feel like you have been researching the best dieting plan.) And you *will* spend time with the subject if you have the disease or are a practitioner trying to help those who do.

Unfortunately, there are no decent, nontechnical books on Lyme disease or its treatment and very few decent technical ones. A comprehensive technical work that includes an overview of the thousands of studies that have been published is desperately needed. And while there are a number of popular press books intended for the lay reader, none of them are particularly good from a treatment perspective. Those that do exist are generally written by people in one of three categories: those who have fought the medical system to force a recognition their condition, conservative medical practitioners outlining conservative treatment protocols, or a very few, badly written books on alternative approaches. Only the microbiologists are uninvolved in the Lyme wars and while their work is remarkable and enlightening to read, it is expensive, highly technical, and, often, slow going.

Whether I actually am or not, I will be perceived as taking sides in the Lyme wars by the writing of this book. You should understand up front that many conservative physicians will not agree with some of the material in this book; in fact, some may disagree almost violently with it. A number of alternative practitioners will have trouble with it as well, and perhaps for similar reasons—their agenda is just different than that of conservative physicians. The nonfundamentalist, middle ground is a lonely place to be in the first decade of the twenty-first century.

I began my examination of Lyme disease without preconceptions, motivated by a desire (as I still am) to understand the organism, the disease it causes, and a wish to sensibly expand the scope of treatment options. I am used to examining interesting diseases and I expected to find a lot of research material on Lyme, which I did. I did expect that nonpharmaceutical approaches to treatment would not be included in mainstream medical practice; that is a given in the United States. And this, too, I did find to be true. What I did not expect to find is that a significant amount of reputable research is being ignored by the mainstream medical community. But that, too, I did find and it troubles me considerably. Science, though it often is, should never be the plaything of the powerful nor used to control the innocent for the accumulation of power and profit. It is through this perversion of science that science and its practitioners lose the credibility they must have for science to continue to be used effectively in this world.

In this book, I will tell you as clearly as I can what my own biases and perspectives are and what I have found from an extensive review of the Lyme literature, whether that be scientific, the writings of physicians and herbalists on the front lines, or the extensive material compiled by those who suffer the disease themselves. What I have found in the scientific literature differs in some important respects from many conservative medical proclamations about Lyme disease.

Six points stand out to me after a rather long and intense examination of the existing material: (1) There is a lot of hysteria about Lyme disease. Everybody is pretty scared, most are not really sure what to do, including the physicians; (2) There are a lot more sick people than the statistics indicate; (3) Antibiotics are not nearly as effective as purported to be; (4) Clear, concise, unemotional information is hard to obtain; (5) Tests for Lyme disease are not very reliable; (6) Something very strange is going on in the field of Lyme disease and its treatment.

I will talk more about these in different sections of the book but I will touch on three of the issues here: rates of infection in the United States; the mode of transmission of the disease; and the effectiveness of antibiotics.

Firstly, it is continually stated by the media and in many medical reports that, in the United States, only about 20,000 people are infected with Lyme disease each year. This figure comes from the Centers for Disease Control (CDC), and is based on the reporting criteria that the CDC has established for the disease. It is crucial to realize that the criteria used to report incidence of the disease is NOT the same as the diagnostic criteria used by physicians. Even though a physician determines that a patient has Lyme disease and successfully treats it with antibiotics, he cannot report it to the CDC if the reporting criteria set by the CDC are not met by the disease symptoms and test results for that particular patient. This difference between diagnostic criteria and reporting criteria is alone responsible for much of the highly incorrect information being disseminated by the press in the United States about infection rates.

Beyond this, there are also numerous problems with the CDC criteria *as reporting criteria* alone, not the least of which is that borrelia organisms are many times present in very small numbers in the body, are often sequestered in hard to reach places, and antibodies are sometimes low enough in infected individuals that they do not show in blood tests for the disease. In other words, people can be, and often are, infected, and the tests generally used for the disease may not show any presence of the bacteria. Numerous studies have shown that the use of more sensitive tests by more highly trained clinicians find that many people, previously pronounced seronegative, in fact, have had Lyme disease all along.

Further, no matter the reason for it, an in-depth analysis of the data reveals that the 20,000 figure is, and has been all along, horribly underrepresentative of actual infection rates in the United States. To get an idea of how much so, Germany, in 1992, reported 30,000 Lyme infections. The population of Germany is about one third that of the United States. A simple extrapolation from Germany's infection rates would put infection rates in the United States at 90,000. This is the lowest figure that should be used in estimating the numbers of Lyme infections in the U.S. each year. This, too, is probably conservative. A number of different researchers, at Harvard and elsewhere, after having examined the data, put the number of yearly infections more in the neighborhood of 200,000.

> *Epidemiologic data suggest that the actual incidence of Lyme disease could be as much as 10 times higher than CDC data indicate. This probably is a result of a restrictive case definition from the CDC, inevitable misdiagnosis, and the fact that physicians tend to underreport reportable diseases of all kinds.*
>
> —JONATHAN EDLOW, M.D.,
> Harvard Medical School

Secondly, the disease is believed to be spread by ticks alone. Regrettably, this assertion is incorrect. Although tick transmission appears to be, and probably is, the primary route of human infection, little research has been conducted on other routes of transmission.

Research has found infectious Lyme spirochetes, for example, in human breast milk, tears, urine, and semen. The disease has also been shown to have been transmitted to babies in the womb. And, finally, live spirochetes have been found in mosquitos, mites, fleas, and biting flies and transmission through some of these routes has been documented. The conventional medical insistence that transmission occurs through ticks alone has stalled research into other modes of transmission and the rates of transmission that are occurring through them. And these other routes may play a much greater role than is currently recognized.

For instance, Lyme spirochetes invade the urinary bladder of all mammals they infect and live spirochetes are commonly expressed in urine of infected animals. Although this route of infection has not been explored, it should be mentioned that leptospira spirochetes, closely related organisms, infect other animals primarily through this route. The tendency for the spirochetes to heavily infect just this organ and to pass live out of the body through the urine is not happenstance. Organisms with the length of survival history as Lyme spirochetes do not "accidentally" colonize the urinary bladder and "accidentally" get expressed out of the body in urine. It is a mechanism of both survival and transmission that is common among many bacteria, because it works and it works very well.

To take it a bit further, when they are "starved," Lyme spirochetes undergo alterations in their physical form. They change into an encysted form from which they can emerge when conditions improve. Ninety-five percent of starved spirochetes can encyst within one minute of expression. These encysted forms have been shown to remain viable for as long as ten months. Other types of spirochetes have been shown to be viable up to two and a half years after encysting. Lyme spirochetes in their encysted form have been shown to survive both freezing and thawing and still be capable of infecting test animals. Because of the constant urination of infected animals, these encysted forms of the organism liberally cover the soil and plants in areas where Lyme disease is endemic. Animals that then take these encysted forms inside themselves through browsing can be infected by viable spirochetes. Lyme spirochetes do live in the intestinal tract quite well and can spread from there throughout the body. Reconversion to motile forms begins within one hour though it has taken up to 6 weeks for full reconversion in some studies. There is significant potential for spirochete transmission in urine.

Also, Lyme spirochetes are masters of collagen tissues—they travel through them easier than they do through blood. Transmission via semen into and then through vaginal tissues is something that is exceptionally easy for Lyme spirochetes. While no one has examined this in detail, studies have found that the rates of infection among married couples is significantly higher than statistical averages would indicate. It has been assumed that this occurs because both people live in a similar tick-heavy environment. Assumptions like that are dangerous in these kinds of situations.

And finally, antibiotics are believed to be highly effective in treating Lyme disease and for many people they are. I do wish to stress this: *for many people they are.* The turnaround in symptoms for many very ill people who take antibiotics is, in fact, (no other word is appropriate here) miraculous. People have gone from being wheel-chair-bound and incapacitated as to any normal life, to fully functional after a proper diagnosis and a course of antibiotics. Unfortunately, an in-depth review of the literature reveals that antibiotics are not nearly as effective as they are purported to be. Studies show that the effectiveness rates for antibiotics run anywhere from 70%-95% depending on the study. Rarely included in these statistics, however, is the fact that there is often as much as a 35% relapse rate. Additionally, live spirochetes are regularly found in people who have been on antibiotic therapy for years or who have undergone repeated, very potent, antibiotic regimens. The Lyme organism is highly adaptable and is able, in a large minority of instances, to evade antibiotic regimens, even those of long duration. Continual antibiotic dosing can and does keep the organisms at low levels in the body, but studies regularly show that it does not eradicate them in up to 40% of those who are treated. The longer a Lyme infection is untreated, the greater chance that it will not respond to antibiotic therapy. Given the difficulty of diagnosis (the characteristic bull's-eye rash only appears in about one third of those bitten by ticks) and the serious under-reporting of infection rates, the numbers of those who are treated within one month of infection is low. After this time period (one week to one month), the disease becomes progressively harder to eradicate.

I admit to a bias. In general, I am not a fan of antibiotics and I have written about their overuse and antibiotic-resistance problems in two previous books—in most detail in *The Lost Language of Plants*. Antibiotics, like many pharmaceuticals, are horribly overused in the United States and, in spite of what medical advertisers say, our health as a nation is not the better for it. We are far down on the list of the industrialized nations in both life expectancy and our quality of life. Antibiotic resistance among some very dangerous organisms is a growing problem because of the continual improper use of antibiotics in the U.S. And, in spite of regular alerts from such organizations as the CDC, nothing seems able to slow that use in either hospitals or among physicians. My standard criteria for antibiotic use, very different than the majority of physicians, is that they should not be used except in instances where there is a high chance of death or disability. Otherwise, we are soon likely not to have them as a treatment option at all. And that has ramifications that few of us really wish to contemplate.

There are several potential reasons for antibiotic treatment failure in LB. One of the possible causes is the persistence of borreliae in tissues.

—G. STANEK, et al.
"History and Characteristics
of Lyme Borreliosis"

However, the level of disability that can occur during Lyme infection makes the use of antibiotics warranted in this disease (even by my criteria). Again, antibiotics are spectacularly effective for many people. This does not mean they work for everyone or even a large majority of people who use them. It is, in part, that failure of effectiveness that drives the need for alternatives that are well considered and that can help in the treatment of the disease. There is a reason so many Lyme sufferers seek out alternative treatments. It is not because they are insane, uneducated, overly hysterical, stupid, or gullible. It is because they are ill, they know they are ill, and because conventional medical treatment has not worked for them. Too often, when they turn to their physicians for help after antibiotics fail, they are told it is all in their heads, or that they will just have to live with their reduced functionality, or that they actually are better—they just can't tell. And unfortunately, many find themselves in the middle of the Lyme wars where the paradigm of treatment becomes more important than the health and happiness of the patients themselves.

The best, short, in-depth analysis of the problems with current Lyme disease diagnosis and treatment (and what the research really shows about the organism) that comes from a clear, concise, scientific, perspective can be found in the article "Lyme disease: ancient engine of an unrecognized borreliosis pandemic?" by W. T. Harvey and P. Salvato (*Medical Hypothesis* 2003;60(5), 742-759). The authors examined nearly a thousand peer-reviewed papers and books on Lyme disease and its treatment for the article. They are researchers as well as physicians and both have had extensive experience with the disease and its treatment.

For those who are interested I include as well an extensive list of sources in the reference section at the end of this book.

CHAPTER ONE

Borrelia Burgdorferi: a Potent Emerging Disease

❦

Compared to what we know about other bacteria that cause disease, our information concerning the spirochetes is by far quite minimal.
—CHUNHAO LI, et al.

Lyme disease is caused by a particular kind of bacterium—a spirochete. Spirochetes are some of the most ancient bacteria on Earth; they have been around billions of years longer than humans and they are very smart. The word *spirochete* literally means "coiled hair." And while this does describe their appearance to some extent, they actually look, more than anything else, like a tiny, very active, worm.

There are eight different genera or kinds of spirochetes: *Borrelia, Brachyspira, Brevinema, Cristispira, Leptonema, Leptospira, Spirochaeta, Treponema.* Over 200 different species in these eight genera have been identified so far, and there are quite likely thousands more. New ones, like the not-yet-formally-named "*Spironema culicis*" recently isolated from mosquitos, are being found all the time. The ability of new-to-science spirochetes like these to infect human beings is still unknown. It is suspected that diseases from so-far-undiscovered spirochetes are the cause of a number of common human ailments for which no known agent has yet been identified.

But not all spirochetes are dangerous to human health. Many types are essential coevolutionary partners of other life forms; they live quite happily in a wide variety of intestinal tracts, including those of humans. Some of the more interesting (up to 20 different kinds) live in the termite gut where they help process the wood fibers that termites eat. All of these different spirochetes, the helpful and the disease-causing, descended from a common spirochetal ancestor billions of years ago.

The kind of spirochetes that cause Lyme disease belong to the genus *Borrelia*. The way Latin terminology works is that the first name—of a bacteria or a plant, for instance—is the genus name, the second is the species name. The organism that causes most of the Lyme disease in the United States is called *Borrelia burgdorferi* (though there are a few caveats about that which I will get to in a minute). *Borrelia* is the genus, *burgdorferi* the species or rather, the particular kind of borrelia that we are talking about. Sometimes for ease, this Latin terminology is abbreviated *B. burgdorferi* or even, in the case of Lyme disease, *Bb*.

To make it all more complicated there are actually a number of borrelia organisms that infect people. Some of these are pretty straightforward when it comes to their naming. For example, *Borrelia hermsii* and 14 other closely related types of borrelia cause what is called "relapsing fever." They are generally named for the species of vector or tick they live within. So the species of *Borrelia* and the species of tick have the same species name. With *Borrelia hermsii* the vector is the tick *Ornithodoros hermsii*. All of the *Borrelia* named like this cause a type of relapsing fever of one sort or another or rather, more correctly, relapsing fever borreliosis. Unfortunately, the borrelia organisms that cause Lyme disease are not named so straightforwardly. All of them do cause Lyme borreliosis (for want of a better term) but the terminology involved is rather inelegant and clunky.

There are three main *Borrelia* that are considered to be the cause of Lyme borreliosis: *Borrelia burgdorferi*, *B. afzelii*, and *B. garinii*. But while these are the main organisms that have been identified so far, more are being found all the time and these others can, and do, cause human infection from time to time. Additional species that have been identified are: *B. lonestari*, *B. valaisiana*, *B. andersonii*, *B. japonica*, *B. lusitanie*, *B.*

turdae, B. tanukii, B. spielmani, and *B. bissettii.* Because these different borrelia organisms cause a Lyme-type infection (just as other borrelia organisms cause infections of the relapsing fever type) they are considered to be part of the Lyme borreliosis grouping. This group of Lyme-type disease organisms is referred to (ridiculously) as *Borrelia burgdorferi sensu lato* (*sensu lato* meaning "in the broad sense"). This is sometimes abbreviated *Bbsl.* The original *B. burgdorferi,* when it is being talked about specifically, is often referred to as *Borrelia burgdorferi sensu stricto* (*sensu stricto* meaning "in the strict sense"). This is sometimes abbreviated *Bbss.* And to make it even more complicated, there are numerous subspecies. Lyme borrelia organisms can rapidly change their genetic structures in response to environmental pressures. This produces slight alterations in the types of borrelia organisms that are found. These are sometimes identified as well, e.g. *Borrelia burgdorferi sensu stricto strain B31.* And to take it even farther, the other Lyme borrelia are sometimes referred to as, for instance, *Borrelia burgdorferi subspecies afzelii,* as if there were not enough confusion already.

Borrelia burgdorferi is considered to be the primary agent of Lyme borreliosis in the United States while *B. afzelii* and *B. garinii* are considered to be the primary agents of European and Asian Lyme disease. Very simplistically, *B. burgdorferi* is considered to be the primary cause of Lyme arthritis, *B. afzelii* of dermatoborreliosis (severe Lyme skin disease), and *B. garinii* of neuroborreliosis (central nervous system Lyme disease). This is, like many definitive statements about Lyme disease, overly simplistic and often incorrect. *B. burgdorferi* is more common in the United States, the others more common in Europe and Asia but all (and many others besides) exist on all three continents and infections with more than one type of Lyme spirochete commonly occur. All of them are able to cause markedly different symptom pictures at different times in different people in different places. They are not limited to specific continents. All borrelia organisms are moving around the world with a great deal of freedom—airplanes are used by more life forms than just people. The other types of Lyme borrelia listed above, although not as common as the three main types, have also been found to cause human infection on various continents and in various combinations. It seems likely that the number of borrelia organisms that cause Lyme borreliosis will eventually, like those that cause relapsing fever, be seen as one related group that cause a similar infection picture.

All of the borrelia species are pathogenic, that is, they all cause disease. And while many types of spirochetes live wild in Nature, no borrelia species have been found to do so. They always seem to need a host species in which to live. All the *Treponema* spirochetes are similar in this respect, though they are better known for causing syphilis (*Treponema pallidum*), yaws (*Treponema pertenue*), and periodontal disease (*Treponema denticola*).

Lyme spirochetes resemble nothing so much as a corkscrew-shaped worm, which is what they act like when they enter living tissues. They literally "screw" or "worm" their way through tissues to the sites they wish to colonize. This kind of mobility allows them to colonize highly viscous mediums such as the collagenous tissues around the knees or the aqueous humor of the eye. Free-living spirochetes, the ones that do live apart in Nature, like to live in similar substances, usually thick mud. Non-spirochetal bacteria enjoy more liquid mediums; they cannot easily exist in the kinds of viscous environments that spirochetes prefer. But spirochetes are highly mobile organisms and they seek these kinds of thick mediums in which to live. It is part of their makeup. Among borrelia organisms, over 6% of their genome structure is dedicated to motility factors. This means that a huge amount (relatively speaking) of their genetic code is designed to implement the unique and powerful movement characteristics that these spirochetes have.

Spirochetes are difficult organisms for researchers to work with, which is why so little (bacterially-speaking) is known about them. They are what is called "fastidious" organisms, meaning that they do

The common morphological structure of spirochetes allows these organisms to bore through highly viscous gel-like media, such as connective tissues, which inhibit the motility of most other bacteria . . . Leptospira *and other spirochetes increase their speed in media with a higher viscosity.*

—Chunhao Li, et al.
"Gyrations, Rotations, Periplasmic Flagella: The Biology of Spirochete Motility"

not like to grow in laboratories and they are real particular about what they eat. The syphilis spirochete, even after sixty years of focused research and antibacterial treatment, still cannot be grown in a laboratory. So special, and difficult-to-manage, growth mediums are used for those that will grow in laboratories. Spirochetes are not your any-old-bacteria that will grow on any-old-piece of toast at the drop of a hat. They are also very thin and this makes them hard to see in microscopes without unusual lighting or specific and expensive kinds of equipment. And, finally, they grow very slowly. Unlike many bacteria that produce a new generation every twenty minutes, Lyme spirochetes do so every 8-12 hours. These three factors alone (and there are others) have made it very hard to do research on spirochetes and the Lyme spirochete is no exception.

The too-oft-told story of Lyme disease is that it was first discovered (and named) when an unusual cluster of what was thought to be juvenile arthritis occurred in Lyme, Connecticut, in the United States, in 1975. A significant number of both children (and adults) in the closely located communities of Lyme, Old Lyme, and East Haddam, Connecticut, were found to have a unique form of juvenile inflammatory arthritis. The incidence of infection in these children was, it was found, 100 times the national average.

The researchers involved in studying the disease decided that it was an unusual form of juvenile arthritis, one that was probably caused by bacteria since the administration of penicillin tended to shorten the course of the disease. They named it Lyme arthritis (unfortunately), after the town. Then in 1982, the researcher Willy Burgdorfer, an expert in spirochetal diseases, discovered a previously unidentified spirochete in ticks on Long Island, New York. The spirochetes reacted with the

> *The pathogenic spirochetes are notoriously difficult to work with. They tend to be difficult or unable to grow* in vitro. *The spirochete growth or maintenance media are generally very complex, time consuming to prepare, and costly. The pathogenic spirochetes also have a propensity to be very fragile and are therefore easily disrupted by standard manipulations.*
>
> —HARDHAM and ROSEY,
> "Antibiotic Selective Markers and Spirochete Genetics"

serum from people in Lyme, Connecticut and the causative agent of Lyme arthritis was found. The disease was renamed Lyme disease and the spirochete named *Borrelia burgdorferi* in honor of Willy Burgdorfer. In actual fact, the disease is more properly called Lyme borreliosis (again, for want of a better term) and I will try to call it that throughout the rest of the book.

It is often said that Lyme borreliosis is an emerging disease (true) and that it is a fairly recent one (false). Lyme borreliosis is an emerging disease in that it is a growing and serious health threat throughout the temperate world (and possibly elsewhere). It is currently the most common vector-borne disease in the United States. The impacts of the disease are often serious and the number of people who are infected continues to rise each yaer. However, it is not accurate to say that it is a new disease.

※

Spirochetes represent an evolutionarily discrete cul-de-sac, forming a relatively close-knit group of organisms that, based on 16S RNA analyses, diverged from other bacteria during early evolutionary history.

—Saier and Paulsen,
"Whole Genome Analyses of
Transporters in Spirochetes: *Borrelia burgdorferi* and *Treponema pallidum*"

While the earliest accounts of the disease in the medical literature date from the late 1880s, and examination of tick specimens from the late 1800s do show that Lyme borreliosis was present in ticks at that time, it is unlikely that the pathogen first infected people during that era. Genomic analysis shows that Lyme spirochetes long ago split off as unique organisms, at a minimum some 100 million years ago. Lyme borrelia have been well-established in ticks and other vectors for a very long time; they do not exist in the wild nor without a host. So for some 100 million years Lyme disease spirochetes have lived in vectors like ticks and they have regularly infected mammals, and lizards, and birds—pretty much anything a tick can get away with biting. It is, in fact, impossible that they had not come into contact with human beings until the late nineteenth century. Lyme borreliosis, like the ticks and the spirochetes themselves, has been with us a very long time.

Recent research suggests that Lyme infection was common in the

Louisiana Tchefuncte Indians between 500 BCE and 300 CE. As well, the heavy presence and complexity in the genomic variety of Lyme borreliosis species in Vladivostok in northeast Asia suggests transfer across Siberia into Alaska between 30,000 BCE and 10,000 BCE. The prevalence and unique genome alterations of the primary American borrelia organism, *Borrelia burgdorferi*, in Europe also suggests spread from the Americas after the heavy European contact that began in 1492.

Borrelia burgdorferi sensu lato has been around a long time and it has infected people for a long time. It was just not possible until very recently to isolate the organism, to see it under a microscope, or to grow it in a laboratory. The litany of symptoms that the organism causes, for example, arthritis and neurological complications, have been with the human species for millennia. Many of these conditions have, until now, been considered idiopathic, that is, from no known cause.

So while it is not true that this is a new disease to human beings, what *is* true is that the agents of Lyme borreliosis are undergoing rapid change. The recent history of Lyme borrelia organisms, as researchers have commented, has been genetically turbulent, showing that the bacteria and their "plasmids are currently in a state of rapid evolutionary change." Like many pathogenic bacteria, the spirochetes that cause borreliosis are feeling tremendous environmental pressure from the massive environmental alterations and antibiotic usage that currently accompany human civilization. They are altering themselves very quickly in response to these pressures and the human species is feeling the impacts.

The Uniqueness of Borrelia

Borrelia organisms are unique in the microbial world. They possess features unusual to bacteria (prokaryotes), features that are more often associated with what are called eukaryotes (more complex, non-bacterial life forms like ticks and people). Unlike nearly all other bacteria, they have, as researchers Saier and Paulsen comment, "linear chromosomes, a cytoskeleton, and periplasmic flagelli that confer rapid motility and unusual chemotactic properties." Borrelia are so unusual, in fact, that they were initially classified with protozoa, not bacteria. They are also unique in that they possess the largest number of genetic units of replication (DNA replicons) of any bacteria known, making them by far the most complex in this respect. They are also among the extremely low number of organisms that have evolved to not require iron in order to live. Too, the borrelia spirochetes have no very close relatives. The closest are probably the *Treponema* spirochetes, the same ones that cause syphilis. But even they only show about a 40% similarity in genome structure to the Lyme borrelia.

While heretical, in many respects Lyme borrelia organisms can (and possibly should) be thought of as an intermediate life form between bacteria and more complex parasites, having the qualities of both. While this is outside conventional thinking, it automatically engenders a better understanding of the organism's behavior during infection. For Lyme spirochetes act like nothing so much as an exceptionally intelligent protozoal parasite. Borrelia organisms are parasitic, and must be thought of as such, because of the way their metabolism is structured. They are capable of only minimal metabolism and all nucleotides, amino acids, fatty acids, and enzyme cofactors must be scavenged from their hosts. This is a primary reason they cannot live in the wild. Unfortunately for us, Lyme spirochetes also have the flexibility of bacteria in that they can rapidly rearrange their gene structure. They do this in order to hide from antibiotics and to better fit themselves into new host animals like humans, while at the same time avoiding their immune systems.

Borrelia Tick Vectors and Animal Hosts

Lyme spirochetes, as I mentioned in the introduction, are passed not only through tick bites but also through other mechanisms. Once they infect people they can be found in breast milk, in tears, in semen, and in urine. Babies have been infected through their mothers while in the womb. Regrettably, little research has been done on the amount of transmission through these kinds of media, the focus has been on ticks. In spite of this limitation, what has been discovered so far is remarkable. The life cycle of *Borrelia* spirochetes, how they live in insect and arthropod vectors (like ticks), and how they infect animals truly is amazing.

Borrelia organisms are considered to be transmitted mainly by particular kinds of ticks, members of the *Ixodes* genera. In the northeastern and middle United States, the primary species is *Ixodes scapularis* (formerly called *Ixodes dammini*). In the western and southern U.S. it is *Ixodes pacificus*. In Europe it is *Ixodes ricinus*, and in Asia it is *Ixodes persulcatus*. This is what you will see in the literature if you study it at all, and it is true that these tick vectors do, in fact, act to transmit the disease and they are probably the primary vectors. What is unclear is how many other vectors are involved in Lyme borreliosis transmission and there are a lot of possible candidates.

B. burgdorferi sensu lato has been found in a at least twenty-five different *Ixodes* species and in fifteen other kinds of ticks including species of *Amblyomma, Boophilus, Dermacentor, Haemaphysalis, Hyalomma, Rhipicephalus, Argas,* and *Ornithodoros.* Lyme spirochetes have also been found in biting flies, mites, fleas, and mosquitos. Transmission to humans has been documented from biting flies (Connecticut and Germany) and from mites (Russia), and is considered to have occurred from mosquitos through mechanical transfer (e.g., squashing a feeding mosquito on the arm). Direct mosquito transfer has not been established but there is every reason to expect that it does occur.

Borrelia spirochetes are very durable in mosquitos and infection rates are moderate to high in some areas. Research has also found that the spirochetes can be transmitted generationally from adult mosquitos through their eggs and that those spirochetes do survive in the newly hatched larvae. Lyme spirochetes have also been found to survive mosquito overwintering. Although the number of spirochetes tend to be lower in mosquitos than in ticks, the spirochetes are well established in them. Regular transmission through alternative routes such as mosquitos, mites, and biting flies, although lower than that of ticks, does occur.

Lyme spirochetes have been found to infect dogs, cats, horses, cows, goats, pigs, sheep, and chickens but they really only like dogs and horses. And while infections in both have become a serious problem, Lyme spirochetes like wild hosts the best. The ticks that carry *Borrelia* spirochetes attach themselves to over 300 different species of mammals, birds, and reptiles. The spirochetes easily transmit to many if not all of these. Over 60 bird species are known to harbor infected ticks and they are important hosts for the spirochetes. Birds, because of the long distances they travel, are responsible for some of the wide dissemination of the disease. And although Lyme borreliosis is considered to be primarily a northern-latitude disease, increasing numbers of infections are being found in such places as Australia, northern and southern Africa, Mexico, the Caribbean, and South America. In Peru, two percent of agricultural workers have been found to be seropositive for the disease.

The Borrelia/Tick Relationship

Borrelia infection has been looked at for too long as simply another disease, like mumps or measles, but it is not. It is considerably more complex. While all diseases are expressions of the ecology of the planet, Lyme borreliosis, more than most, intimately pulls each of us—those who wish to understand it, treat it, or are infected by it—into interconnected webs of ecological complexity. Borrelia is different than other diseases.

Borrelia have host-parasite interactions that are basically different from the more well understood pathogens.

—SHERWOOD CASJENS,
"Borrelia Genomes"

Many bacteria are looked at in a linear fashion, with a starting point and an end point. With Lyme borrelia that is a difficult approach for there is no one starting point, no one end point. It is a very circular organism and any place that you begin is arbitrary.

The ixodes ticks that carry Lyme spirochetes have three stages of growth—larval, nymph, and adult—and each stage only feeds once. When they are engorged, filled with the blood meal from their host, they drop off, digest their meal, and either moult into a new stage or, in the case of the adults, lay eggs for a new generation.

Basically, Lyme ticks, of whatever species, are not very mobile, they have been found to be able to move on their own only about nine feet (three meters) from where they hatch or drop off after feeding. They basically just sit there until something with blood comes by. Then they hitch a ride.

The ticks that cause most of the Lyme borreliosis in the northeastern United States give a fairly good picture of the life cycle of Lyme ticks throughout the world.

The adult ticks lay their eggs in the very early spring and the larvae hatch from them in the summer. It takes about a month for the eggs to hatch once the temperature warms enough. The transmission of Lyme spirochetes to the eggs is low, though it does occur. About one percent of the hatched larvae are usually infected, though up to a fourth of them have been found to be so in some studies. When spirochete transmission to the eggs does occur, viable spirochete levels in the eggs are generally 100%. Although larval transmission of Lyme disease to humans and other mammals is uncommon, it does occur.

Peak larval activity occurs in August. Larval ticks are tiny, about the size of the point of a pin or the period at the end of this sentence. Impossible to see really. After they hatch, they attach to a host and begin to feed. They like smaller animals, those closer to the ground, such as mice.

As soon as larvae (or any growth stage of these ticks) start to feed, they begin releasing a unique blend of chemicals into the blood stream of their host. Among other things these act as potent chemical cues for any spirochetes that happen to be in the animal they are now feeding upon. Once tick saliva factors are sensed, existent spirochetes immediately enter the blood stream and flow to the site of larval attachment. This is important since most larvae are not infected with spirochetes at birth. Once the larvae start feeding, spirochetes flow through the bloodstream and then enter the previously uninfected tick larva in its blood meal. Thus the disease passes on into a new generation. Once they enter the new tick, the spirochetes primarily colonize the tick gut tissues.

Ticks contain what is called *TROSPA*. It is a special tick receptor (TR) that binds to proteins in the outer surface (or skin) of the spirochetes' bodies. This outer surface protein (denoted Osp, type A or OspA) attaches to the tick receptor (TROSPA) in the tick gut allowing colonization to occur. This works in many respects like iron-filings and a magnet. The spirochetes are pulled toward the TROSPA in the tick gut and stick. Once they are attached to the tick gut tissues, the Lyme spirochetes may go on to infect many other sites within the tick: the hypodermis, central ganglion, salivary glands, ovaries, and connective tissues.

The larval tick, when it is done feeding, drops off the animal it has been on wherever the animal happens to be. Larvae generally feed for 72 hours, or about three days, before becoming engorged and dropping off. Once they drop off they absorb their blood meal and begin to moult, to change form into the next stage of tick development, called the nymph. This takes about 35 days on average. The newly emerged nymphs winter over and begin their activity the next spring. Many nymphs carry Lyme spirochetes due to infection of the larval-stage tick during its life cycle. The number of new nymphs that are infected depends on many things, from what kind of winter it was to the density of mice in the area that particular year. Infection rates have been found to run anywhere from 3% to 100%. Generally, in endemic areas, at least half of all nymphs are infected with Lyme spirochetes at the beginning of the season. More are infected as that season progresses due to the spirochetes responsiveness to tick saliva factors during multiple nymph attachments.

The nymph is bigger than the larva but still horribly small, about the size of the head of a pin. They are generally hard to see when not engorged with a blood meal. Nymphs begin their activity in May and are very active through the summer. They will feed on pretty much anything that they can, from mice to people. The nymphs are highly infective and so, by the time the larvae hatch and begin *their* peak activity, most animals in a Lyme endemic area will be infected. Many will still have nymphs attached. This overlap in the tick cycle ensures that many if not most larvae will be infected before they moult.

Nymphs feed longer than larvae—four or five days. When they are engorged they drop off and begin to moult into adult ticks. This takes a bit longer than the larval moult, about 42 days on average. For all stages of tick—larva, nymph, or adult—it may take days or weeks to digest the single blood meal it has taken.

The adult ticks emerge from moult in October or early November and they immediately begin looking for a meal. They are larger than either larvae—or nymph—stage ticks; they look about the same as any old tick you might have seen. Often they climb to the tops of stalks of grass or other plants and wait, their upper legs stretched out, for a passing animal to brush against them so they can hitch a ride. Adult ticks are more discriminatory in their feeding habits than when in other stages of growth, they like larger animals such as deer, horses, dogs, and people. They tend to not feed on anything smaller than a woodchuck or dog. They also feed much longer—seven or eight days. Once they are full they, too, drop off and prepare themselves to overwinter. Some adult ticks, those that have not found a host to feed from in the fall, overwinter and try to feed in the spring. Both fall-fed and spring-fed ticks lay their eggs in the spring, anywhere from two to three thousand of them per tick, and then they die. If winters are especially warm, they may emerge from hibernation and feed at any time.

The eggs they lay take about a month to hatch. Lucky for us, there is an exceptionally large egg and larval mortality. Both are fed upon by a number of predatory insects and arthropods such as ants, spiders, and wasps. Birds eat a great many of the ticks as well, often before the ticks lay their eggs.

Ticks that transmit Lyme spirochetes do live in warmer climates such as the American south, the American west coast, northern Africa, and southern Europe. Their particular growth patterns differ from ticks that are limited by colder winters such as those from the American northeast. Their life cycles can run anywhere from two to six years. And unfed ticks are remarkably patient, some of them can live up to five years without a meal.

The population levels of the ticks that carry Lyme spirochetes are increasing and the ticks are constantly moving into new areas. This is

With Ixodes dammini, *the birth rate clearly exceeds the death rate over most of its range. Populations of* I. dammini *seem to be increasing in density in areas where they are already established, and there is considerable evidence that the range of this species is expanding both in the Northeast and upper Midwest… Nowhere does there seem to be a trend for a population decline of this species. It is likely that this situation will continue for the immediate future, as* I. dammini *has all the characteristics of an invading species.*

—Durland Fish,
"Population Ecology of *Ixodes dammini*"

directly because of human environmental perturbations. Although the ticks can feed on over 300 different kinds of animals, two of the most important in the northeastern United States are the white-footed mouse and deer. Human destruction of large mammal predators such as mountain lions and panthers have led to the rapid increase in deer herds. Forest cutting has allowed more brush and grasslands to grow, allowing more mice and deer to breed. And overuse of pesticides have killed off large numbers of the predators that feed on tick eggs and larvae, including birds. Climate perturbations that have caused abnormally warm winters and wet summers are also exacerbating the problem. This is expanding tick habitats. All of these factors together have generated tick populations so high in some areas that researchers who dragged a white flannel cloth over a 60-foot (20-meter) section of ground in one study in the United States found 1200 ticks attached. In highly endemic areas, there may be as many as sixty nymphs (on average) feeding on each mouse or fifty adults on each deer. This is the average. Up to 200 nymphs have been found attached to a mouse, 500 on a single deer.

Oversimplistically, the story that is told by most Lyme disease sources (such as government-developed Web sites in the United States) is that nymphs and larvae feed on small animals like white-footed mice. This keeps the spirochete levels in circulation in tick populations. But the adult ticks have to feed on something bigger in order to lay their eggs to make new generations of ticks. Mostly it is deer. Humans get involved when they take a walk in the woods. And this is sort of their fault as is building too many homes in the woods and not living in cities. This is sort of true, I guess.

What is more accurate is that the primary reservoir in the northeast United States is the white-footed mouse. It is true as well that virtually all mice born in an endemic area will become infected in a short period of time. However, the primary reservoir for the spirochetes changes from country to country. And reduction of mice simply moves the spirochetes into a new reservoir species. Reduction of deer habitat through cutting results in temporary reductions in ticks but they rebound fairly quickly. Directly reducing deer populations shows the same thing—a short-term reduction in tick numbers with a large rebound shortly thereafter.

Large mammals like deer are not actually necessary to the spread of the disease. Madeira, a subtropical island off the coast of Portugal, has no large mammals yet Lyme spirochetes spread happily through adult tick attachment to two different species of rats. In other parts of Europe the hedgehog is the primary "large" mammal that they use.

There are in fact five forms of *Borrelia burgdorferi sensu lato* in Europe, with three primary vector species and 35 reservoir host species and all are tightly linked together to maintain the disease in the wild. In Japan, 61 strains of *Borrelia burgdorferi sensu lato* have been isolated. Five species of ixodid ticks primarily spread them (though they have been found in 10 other types of ticks as well). The Japanese field mouse is the primary reservoir and the red fox is one of the two "large" mammals that act as hosts for adult ticks.

Reduction of deer will not end the cycle of infection. Neither will the use of tick pesticides. The use of pesticides to kill the ticks does work for awhile, but ticks like other insects and arthropods have a tendency to develop resistance to pesticides as time goes by. Things are much more complicated in real life than they are on government Web sites.

It is most accurate to realize that Lyme spirochetes are opportunistic parasitic organisms with a great deal of intelligence and experience in promulgating themselves in the wild, as they have done for some 100 million years. They infect a variety of biting insects (mostly arthropods, meaning eight-legged ones) and are injected into new hosts through this mechanism. Both the ticks and their animal hosts are essential in the life cycle of the spirochetes (otherwise the spirochetes would just stay in ticks OR the animal hosts but not both). The spirochetes are not particular. Whatever works is what they will do and they are exceptionally good innovators. That humans are one of their usable hosts and have been for a long time can be seen from the fact that the spirochetes possess separate plasmids (DNA strands) just for people. They can weave these into their chromosomal structure, allowing them to infect humans. They have created a software program especially for this purpose.

Nymph-stage ticks feed quite happily on people. In fact, this is where most human infections come from. Larvae feed on people as well, and though the rate of larva to human infection is low the rate of human to larva infection is much higher. (Adult ticks are much more easily found when feeding on people due to their size, and are often removed before they can feed long enough to pass on the spirochetal infection.) Human beings are actively being woven into the ecological network of the disease. We are no different than our dogs in this respect. And humans, along with birds, are now one of the major life forms that spreads the disease out of endemic areas.

Deer maintain a home range of several miles (4 km), while mice tend to remain in an area of about 100 x 100 feet (30 m square). Lyme spirochetes are being spread farther, not only by expanding animal populations that push younger animals out of established ranges, but primarily by bird flight and human/dog travel into and out of endemic areas.

Spirochete Transfer to a New Host:
The Moment of Tick Bite

When a tick carrying Lyme spirochetes attaches itself to an animal and bites into the skin, a unique series of events immediately begins. And these events are intimately connected to the makeup of tick saliva. This was not recognized for a very long time and has contributed to many misunderstandings about the disease. Needle inoculation of lab animals produces a significantly different kind of infection than tick infections do. Studies on needle-infected lab animals tend to be relatively useless in understanding borrelial infections in people.

When a warm-blooded mammal walks by, the dormant tick grabs hold and begins to look for its preferred attachment site (in rodents, this is often the ears). Once found, the tick begins to saw through the outer layer of the skin so that it can reach the blood vessels that lay just below the surface. The tick then secretes a milky cement that hardens around the penetration site. This holds the tick firmly in place and acts as a kind of gasket that prevents loss of blood from the host or leakage of tick saliva from the point of entry. This gasket is composed of unique glycosylated proteins which are very similar in their makeup to collagen and keratin—two of the major components of vertebrate skin.

Under this point of attachment, a tiny pit is gouged out of the blood-vessel-rich dermis, which then fills with blood. Ticks are, in essence, pool feeders. They let the pit fill and then drink at their leisure. This stage of feeding is slow and its length differs for each stage of the tick life cycle. As the tick (larva, nymph, or adult) feeds, its body engorges considerably. When it is finished feeding, it detaches from the host and falls to the ground where it digests the blood meal and, if larval or nymph, begins the moult. The cement core is left behind, embedded in the skin.

During feeding, the tick alternates between taking blood and releasing saliva into the wound. This saliva, from the moment of attachment, as it enters the blood and surrounding tissues, releases into the host body a complex blend of powerful, pharmacologically active compounds. They are designed to counteract the three main host-immune defenses that arise immediately upon the attachment of something like a tick. These are: hemostasis (blood coagulation, platelet aggregation, and vasoconstriction), inflammation, and immunity (innate and acquired). Tick saliva chemicals are highly bioactive. While only a few of the hundreds of chemicals in tick saliva have been identified, many of their bodily targets have been. The antihemostatic compounds inhibit platelet ADP (adenosine phosphate), prostaglandin receptor, prostacyclin receptor, and thrombin. The anti-inflammatory compounds inhibit anaphylatoxins, histamine, and bradykinin. The anti-immune compounds inhibit the alternative pathway of the complement system, neutrophils, splenic T lymphocytes, B lymphocytes, interleukin 2 (IL-2), IL-8, macrophages, nitric oxide, interferon alpha, interferon gamma, and immunoglobulin G (IgG). This broad range of anti-immune activity has a potent impact on host-immune defense. To get a very brief idea, IgG plays an important role in host defense responses to infection. It protects tissues from bacteria, viruses, and toxins. IgG neutralizes bacterial toxins, activates the complement immune response, and enhances phagocytosis (white blood cell activity against disease organisms). And this is only one part of the immune response that is inactivated or inhibited by tick saliva.

The Lyme spirochete takes advantage of the tick's release of these compounds to infect the host. For example, studies have found that if the levels of interleukin-2 and interferon gamma in lab mice are kept high (counteracting the tick saliva chemicals) the rate of infection drops precipitously.

Tick saliva also inactivates one of our most potent innate immunities to disease—the alternative complement system. When we are born we have what is called *innate* immunity. Over time we also *acquire* immunity to diseases with which we have been infected—so-called acquired immunity. One of the most potent elements of our innate immunity is called the complement system. This part of our immune system can be activated through any of three pathways: the classical complement pathway, the lectin pathway, or the alternative complement pathway. Each pathway is useful for dealing with different kinds of microbes. The alternative complement pathway is the part of our innate immunity that can deal with borrelia spirochetes. In fact, Lyme spirochetes cannot gain a foothold in a host with an active complement system where the alternative pathway is uninhibited. The complement system kills them immediately.

Components in tick saliva specifically inhibit this part of our innate immunity. Lyme spirochetes take advantage of the alternative complement-inhibiting factors in tick saliva to seek out unprotected sites in the host body where they can then take root and grow.

Lyme organisms use many parts of the complex biochemical makeup of their tick hosts to facilitate their infection of mammals upon which the tick happens to feed.

The infection of the body by Lyme spirochetes is enhanced as well if the new host already has low immune function. The degree of infection and how severe symptoms become are directly dependent on host-immune strength or weakness. In addition, a healthy host-immune defense also stimulates antibodies to tick saliva and inhibits future tick attachment. Anti-tick-saliva antibodies cause tick rejection before much feeding can take place. The higher the immune response the less able a tick is to attach and feed and the lower the rate of Lyme infection in those who are exposed to an infected tick bite.

Once the tick begins feeding, as the blood from its host enters the tick stomach, the spirochetes undergo an immediate transformation. Ticks are ambient temperature organisms, that is, the temperature of their bodies is the same as the temperature in the forest where they live. The mammal hosts of Lyme spirochetes are warm-blooded. The spirochete must go from an ambient temperature environment to one where the temperature is kept relatively steady, such as the approximately 98.6 degrees Fahrenheit (37 C) in human beings. Lyme spirochetes live in microclimates that are very different from one another. In ixodid ticks, they primarily sequester themselves in the tick's midgut where not only is there an ambient temperature but the pH is alkaline, about 9.5.

When the blood meal enters the tick gut two things immediately occur: an increase in heat and a decrease in pH from 9.5 to around 7.4. When these changes occur, the spirochetes know that the tick is feeding, and the spirochetes prepare to leave the tick host and enter the mammal host. The dramatic increase in temperature and the alteration of pH are essential environmental cues, and they initiate a regulatory cascade in the spirochete that changes its nature considerably.

Along with their central linear chromosomes Lyme spirochetes can have up to 12 linear and 12 circular plasmids, or 24 extra segments of DNA available at any one time. Basically these are extrachromosomal DNA molecules that in total may equal half the length of their central linear chromosome. The incorporation of this extra DNA is driven by environmental cues.

Each of these DNA strands contain information about different mammals that the spirochetes can live within. The borrelia organisms analyze the blood meal, determine what kind of animal the tick is feeding upon and then separate out the requisite strand of DNA which they then weave into their DNA structure so that they can safely infect the source of the tick's meal. These DNA strands contain information about how the spirochete must alter its physiology in order to avoid the new host's immune system. It is a set of operating instructions as it were, which tells the spirochete how to rearrange its biological structure to facilitate entry and infection of the new host.

As soon as the blood meal is analyzed, the spirochetes begin to multiply rapidly, increasing their number three to four times. A great many of them then migrate from the tick midgut to the tick's salivary glands. There they begin altering their physiological structure. This takes some time, that is why the longer the tick feeds, the more chance there is for infection. Ticks that are removed within 24 hours are much less able to transfer the spirochetes to the new hosts, human or otherwise.

Spirochetes are unusual in that they have an inner protein coat and an outer protein coat. *Borrelia* spirochetes are no exception. This two-coat arrangement is something like a hand with a thin latex glove on the outside. It is this outside coat that comes into contact with the host organisms the spirochete lives within. So, for each animal species it learns to infect, the spirochetes maintain a database of information that tells it just how to rearrange that protein coat. These protein coats are referred to by the initials Osp (for outer surface protein), and there are six primary types coded as Osp A-F. There are still others, each coded differently, such as Erp and VlsE.

While in the tick, many of the spirochetes' outer surface protein coats are type A (OspA). After they encounter a blood meal some, but not all, of the spirochetes downregulate OspA and begin to upregulate OspC. This change occurs in a

Many infectious bacteria have limited host ranges, due to their encoding proteins capable of interacting with tissues of only certain hosts. However, for survival in nature, Lyme disease-associated borreliae must be able to infect many different kinds of vertebrate hosts, since many of their tick vectors will feed upon a variety of mammals and birds. Since an infected tick feeds only a limited number of times during its life, a bacterium must be able to seize each opportunity for transmission and ultimately, survival of its lineage. By encoding multiple alleles of infection-associated proteins, each capable of interacting with different potential hosts, there will be an increased chance of efficiently infecting whichever vertebrate the tick vector feeds upon.

—STEVENSON, et al.
"Repetition, Conservation, and Variation:
the Multiple cp32 Plasmids
of *Borrelia* Species"

minority of the spirochetes, less than half. Others upregulate, for example, OspE, or OspF, or Erp (a similar OspE/F protein). These Erp proteins, when they are expressed at the outer coat, can bind to a particular part of the complement immune system called factor H. This helps those spirochetes with that specific outer protein surface to avoid the innate immune response once they enter the new host.

The spirochetes also upregulate virulence factors. In essence the spirochetes open up the armory and gear up for assault. Other substances called decorin-binding proteins are upregulated, too. These proteins are known as adhesins; they bind decorin—a molecule that is associated with collagen type III. This aids the spirochetes in colonizing collagen sites in the new host, most importantly, during the initial infection stage in the skin. Plasminogen (as well as its activator urokinase) binding factors are also upregulated. These help the spirochetes to bind themselves to plasminogen during entry into the new host. Plasminogen is an inactive substance that circulates in the blood. It is converted at need to plasmin (by its activator urokinase), an enzyme that inactivates fibrin, the substance that helps blood clot. By binding decorin to their outer surface (it is like putting on camouflage fatigues), the spirochetes hide themselves from the new host's immune system and facilitate their penetration through endothelial cell layers into new areas of the body.

In all, 154 genes are known to be altered when the spirochetes encounter a tick's blood meal. Seventy-five genes are upregulated, half of them normally stored on plasmids. Seventy-nine are downregulated, 70% of them onto plasmids. Among those that are upregulated are chemotaxis and sensing regulons and proteases capable of modifying the outer protein coat.

In essence the spirochetes, upon being notified that the tick has attached to a new host, put on their assault clothing, apply camouflage, and lock and load their weapons. They then move through the salivary glands of the tick for insertion into the new host. The salivary glands are the primary route of transmission to new hosts.

To enhance survivability, not all the spirochetes alter themselves in the same manner. There is a tremendous antigenic variation among them. That is, the spirochetes alter themselves in a variety of ways to enhance the potential of infection in the new host. Some 37 changes to the outer protein membrane have been found to occur so far.

Borrelia burgdorferi sensu lato spirochetes also, like major antibiotic-resistant bacteria, exchange information with each other (and other bacteria as well). This enhances their ability to evade antibiotics, to be more virulent, and to colonize a wider range of new hosts. They also have a much greater ability for multi-drug efflux than other spirochetes such as the ones that cause syphilis. This means that the spirochetes can cause the drugs designed to kill them to rapidly flow out of their bodies before the drugs can harm them.

Lyme spirochetes are exceptionally good at altering their structure from moment to moment in order to evade host-immune responses and to enhance colonization of different parts of the body. They are, in essence, continually experimenting with alterations in their structure to find those that maximize their survival in host tissues. Researchers have described their capacity in this regard as "nearly inexhaustible" and have noted, importantly, that these alterations occur only *in vivo*, never *in vitro* (test tube), making most of the data collected through *in vitro* studies to be nearly useless.

> *Relapsing fever borreliae contain multiple copies of genes encoding surface proteins designated variable membrane proteins (VMPs)... During vertebrate infection VMP-encoding genes continually recombine into new expression locus, and thus bacteria constantly produce new VMPs that are unrecognized by the host immune system, allowing for persistent infection. Lyme disease spirochetes contain a similar genetic system.*
>
> —STEVENSON, et al.
> "Repetition, Conservation, and Variation:
> the Multiple cp32 Plasmids of
> *Borrelia* Species"

Thus the structure of the Lyme spirochetes is constantly in flux. Researchers have found that when they recovered infectious spirochetes from intentionally infected mice, the spirochetes they get out of the mice are not the same as the ones they put in. They are continually recombining, altering their genome structure and, in consequence, their physical expression. As researchers (Qiu, et al.) recently noted, "Frequent recombination implies a potential for rapid adaptive evolution and a possible polygenic basis of *B. burgdorferi* pathogenicity." And different genomic combinations decidedly do create different symptom pictures in the people infected with Lyme spirochetes.

Lyme Borreliosis in People: The Disease

Borrelia spirochetes have a tremendous and very sophisticated ability to sense the makeup of the environment they live within. They are extremely sensitive to exceptionally tiny alterations in their environments. This refined perception comes, in part, through what is called chemotaxis. That is, the spirochetes are highly responsive to tiny chemical shifts, being attracted to some and repelled by others. They can sense chemicals they need for food (e.g. sugars and fats) and others that are harmful to them (e.g. high oxygen concentrations). They are so sensitive to slight chemical alterations in the body that they can sense, almost immediately, the presence of tick biochemical factors if a tick begins to feed on a host in which they are present. If another tick, one that is not infected, begins to feed on an infected host, many of the Lyme spirochetes that are already there flow into the blood stream. These quickly relocate to the site where the uninfected tick is feeding and they are taken into the new tick via the blood.

Lyme spirochetes can also identify large numbers of different kinds of cells in the host and they adhere to different types to facilitate their movement through the host system. This allows the organisms to seek out their preferred tissue sites—joints, aqueous humor of the eye, the meninges of the brain, and various collagenous sites in the body (such as the skin and knees) and heart tissue. (All of these areas have one thing in common—a lot of collagen. Lyme spirochetes love it.)

Lyme organisms have been found to adhere to cultured endothelial and epithelium cells, differentiated neural cells, brain cells, and glial cells. Typically, Lyme spirochetes live deeper within tissues than other kinds of bacteria. They, in fact, can move much faster in viscous material like collagenous tissues than they can in blood.

Lyme infection, like many chronic conditions, produces an imbalance in the Th1 and Th2 immune complexes. T-helper cells (Th) of the immune system can be separated into two functionally distinct groups, 1 and 2. Th1 lymphocytes are characterized by the production of type 1 cytokines such as Interleukin-2 (IL-2), tumor-necrosis factor-beta (TNF-b) and interferon-gamma (INF-gamma). Th2 lymphocytes produce the cytokines interleukin-4 (IL-4), IL-5, IL-6, IL-10, and IL-13. During Lyme borreliosis a powerful Th1 response is initiated by the host to deal with the infection. This is important because there is some evidence that balancing the Th1/Th2 response can lead to better outcomes during treatment. However, significantly lowering the Th1 response, for example, by inhibiting interferon gamma production worsens outcomes. Lyme arthritis is very severe when IFN-gamma is inhibited. (More on all this later.)

There are considered to be three stages of Lyme disease: early, early-disseminated, and late. Early Lyme disease is considered to occur in the days or weeks after initial infection, early-disseminated to occur weeks to months after infection, and late to occur months to years after initial infection. Early stage is initial infection where there has been little spread of the spirochetes and only a bull's-eye rash exists as a symptom. In early-disseminated, the disease has begun to spread but has not yet become chronically entrenched. Late is when it has penetrated a great many parts of the body and established itself as a chronic disease.

This view is simplistic (and often not very accurate) because the disease's progression is markedly different for each infected person. Late stage can occur in only a few months in some people or take years for others. In part, the reason these stages have been delineated is that treatment is much more effective in early stages of the disease and (sometimes) symptoms are very different. Very few people experience clearly demarcated stages of early, early-disseminated, and late-stage infection. Lyme spirochetes, within days of infection are often already present in both the aqueous humor of the eye and the central nervous system. Early-disseminated and early are identical stages for most people.

The primary distinctions for treatment purposes are nearly always going to be early-disseminated and late stages of the disease. The later treatment occurs the harder it is the get rid of the disease. As time goes by the organisms adapt themselves to the person they are in and adjust to the immune response in that individual. They also alter their geno-type, making their offspring more able to survive in just that particular environment. This makes them much harder to remove and is why treatment therapies at that point tend to be longer and often are with more potent medicines or larger doses.

Because the spirochetes have various subtypes or species, because every human immune system is different, and because the spirochetes go to different sites in different numbers in different people, the symp-toms vary widely. Some people have very few symptoms and the condi-tion tends to self-resolve. Others have, from the beginning, severe symptoms and they resolve only partially or with difficulty even with the strongest antibiotic regimens. Most people fall somewhere in between.

Very generally, *Borrelia burgdorferi sensu stricto* infections tend to be more virulently infective and far more inflammatory to tissues espe-cially in the joints and knees. Lyme arthritis is much more common with this type of borrelia. *B. afzelii* tends to be the primary agent of acrodermatitis chronica atrophicans (ACA), though *B. garinii* can also be involved. *B. garinii* is considered to be the primary cause of most neuroborreliosis. These latter two forms of Lyme spirochetes survive the adaptive immune response to a greater degree and survive in the skin and nervous system in far greater numbers than *B. burgdorferi*.

Dermatoborreliosis: Lyme Expressions in Skin

After the spirochetes enter the human body they begin actively spread-ing throughout the tissues. This is why the *erythema migrans* (EM) or bull's-eye rash that some people get upon being infected grows outward in larger and larger circles as time progresses. It is the sign of the move-ment of the spirochetes through the tissues. While EM has long been considered one of the primary markers for Lyme infection it is not a reli-able diagnostic indicator for all people who are infected. This is because only about a third (37%) of the people who are infected have EM as a symptom. (About 20% of people with dermatoborreliosis will have multiple EM rashes.) And only in about 10% of people with EM can Lyme spirochetes be detected in the bloodstream. When EM rash does occur it is nearly always a confirmatory diagnosis for Lyme infection.

Lyme spirochetes use a great many techniques to facilitate their movement through skin for there are many barriers in these tissues to penetration. Tight junctions interconnect cells in the epithelial and endothelial cell layers which make them impermeable to even small molecules. To facilitate penetration, the spirochetes disrupt or rearrange cell cytoskeletons, break down tissue structures through a number of mechanisms (collagenolytic, fibrinolytic, or proteolytic actions), and inhibit the wound-healing factors that would normally occur. This allows Lyme spirochetes to move into the intracellular junctions between endothelial cells and beneath the monolayers, so-called transendothelial migration. This facilitates spirochetal movement into, and through, the endothelial layers, and thus infection in a new host. And they do this together, as a group. The spirochetes synchronize their actions, creating as a cooperative group the proteins needed for infection to occur. During this process some spirochetes can be found intracellularly within fibroblasts. These are the cells that produce collagen fibers and are present in all connective tissues. Even when antibiotics such as ceftriaxone are present at bacteriocidal levels, spirochetes can sometimes escape the antibiotic by their encapsulation in fibroblasts.

There are three primary forms of dermatoborreliosis or Lyme skin infections: erythema migrans (EM), borrelial lymphocytoma (BL), and acrodermatitis chronica atrophicans (ACA). Lyme spirochetes, even if these symptoms are not present, are commonly present in the skin in various parts of the body.

EM, while unsightly, is generally only a sign of spirochete infection; there are few additional complications from its appearance. The EM lesions vary in size, some are small, others very large (up to 70 cm, but the average size is 16 cm). The lesions are usually round or oval, though triangular and linear forms do, rarely, occur. The rash is usually bright red (sometimes bluish-red) and even-toned in color, though some forms, especially in Europe, will show a central area that clears while the rash itself continues to move outward.

Rarely, a very mild pain, burning, or itching can occur; these tend to be localized to the site of the rash. Other general Lyme symptoms can occur along with its initial appearance—low-grade fever, mild chills, fatigue, and neck stiffness. The rash generally enlarges by a few centimeters per day and usually fades within a few weeks even without antibiotic treatment.

Laboratory examination of the area of the rash will generally find what is called mononuclear infiltrate in the skin. This is composed of lymphocytes, histiocytes, and a variable mixture of plasma cells. The older the lesion, the more plasma cells that are present. Very early lesions will sometimes show neutrophil and eosinophil penetration as well. The blood vessels will generally be dilated.

It is important to note that Lyme borreliosis generates both primary and secondary EM lesions. The primary lesions, which are the ones most people know about, generally present soon after tick bite and have a puncture wound near the center of the lesion. Secondary lesions can occur months to years later. They do not have a central puncture wound, and they can be any place on the body, not just where the tick bite occurred. Secondary lesions are symptoms of late stage Lyme borreliosis; they are difficult to distinguish from the early stage rash and misdiagnosis is common.

Borrelial lymphocytoma (BL) are bluish-red nodules that generally occur on the earlobe in children or the nipple in adults. Normally only nipple BL is painful. Sometimes it is called lymphocytoma cutis or lymphadenosis benigna cutis. During BL there is an accumulation of lymphocytes and other inflammatory cells in a localized region of the skin. There are a number of non-Lyme causes for the condition—vaccinations, tattoos, and jewelry. But Lyme infection, especially in eastern Europe, sometimes causes it. It is much less common than EM or ACA and will often occur with or after the typical EM rash. Rarely, BL will show in other locations—scrotum, nose, upper arm, or shoulder.

Acrodermatitis chronica atrophicans (ACA) is fairly rare in the United States. It tends to be caused by the species of Lyme spirochetes that are more common in Europe and Asia—*B. afzelii* and *B. garinii*. It is considered to be primarily caused by *B. afzelii*. For every 10 cases of

Lyme disease, only one will show ACA as a symptom. (Some studies put it much lower than that—35:1.) More women than men (4:1) seem to develop the condition. It is more frequent in those over age forty, very rare in adolescents, and occurs only occasionally in children.

ACA is almost always a late onset condition in untreated Lyme borreliosis. Although it can develop immediately from an early EM rash, it rarely does so. Generally 6-36 months occur between tick bite and early signs of ACA emergence. Usually a localized swelling is the first sign of the disease—often on one foot, hand, or a finger. ACA is usually unilateral, affecting one side of the body, though occasionally bilateral forms have occurred. There is a progressive, exaggerated reaction to pain in the affected area as the disease progresses. Spontaneous acral pain (i.e., pain in the peripheral parts—limbs, fingers, and so on), paresthesia, dysthesia, and cognitive dysfunction are common. The condition progresses into an inflammatory stage with few to several soft, slowly enlarging cutaneous swellings, often bluish-red in color. Multiple fibrotic nodules also occur and are typical. They are generally localized in the vicinity of joints.

In ACA there is a mononuclear infiltrate that is concentrated around blood vessels. The blood vessels themselves are often dilated. The infiltrate extends between the collagen fibers and is primarily composed of lymphocytes and histiocytes, and clustered plasma cells. This is similar to EM but occurs to a much greater degree. In ACA, there is a long-term spirochete infection in the skin that does not resolve (unlike EM lesions). Live spirochetes have been detected in skin lesions up to 10 years after infection.

In ACA of many years duration, the skin will become thin, atrophic, wrinkled, dry, and translucent. The hair on the affected area is lost, sebaceous and sweat glands decrease in number. Minor bumps and scrapes to the affected area will easily produce large, slowly healing ulcers. There is often peripheral neuropathy, musculoskeletal pains, and underlying joint damage.

Treatment with antibiotics is generally effective in people with ACA though in long-term chronic stages of the disease the symptoms may be only partially reversible. (Herbal regimens can help considerably with this, see chapters three and four.) There are no known cases of ACA that have resolved without treatment.

Lyme Arthritis

Borrelia burgdorferi sensu stricto is the type of Lyme spirochete that most commonly causes Lyme arthritis. Lyme arthritis is much less common in Europe where *B. afzelii* and *B. garinii* are more dominant during infection. However, like most Lyme pronouncements, this tends to be true in general but with many exceptions. *B. garinii* has been found to produce an antibiotic-resistant, difficult-to-treat arthritis in a number of Europeans. And *B. burgdorferi* is increasingly found to be the infectious agent in Europe.

Initial Lyme infection is often accompanied by general aches and pains, especially in the joints and muscles. And while the Lyme spirochetes quickly spread through the body during this period, sometimes reaching the knees within days, the condition called Lyme arthritis generally does not set in for several months after infection. In children, for example, the mean time to onset is 4.3 months. The primary sites for Lyme arthritis are the large joints, especially the knees, though other joints can be affected as can the tendons and bursae. In acute attacks, the affected joint will often be intensely swollen to two, three, or four times its normal size. These attacks, like a number of the symptoms of Lyme infection, occur at periodic intervals, seemingly as the spirochete load and antigenic variation, and, more importantly, immune competence, wax and wane. (Often the attacks wax and wane on about a four-week interval and are often, no one knows why, worse during the full moon.)

Lyme spirochetes upregulate a number of outer coat proteins during movement into and through the human body. A number of these directly affect spirochete presence around the joint and its subsequent inflammation. Of particular note are fibronectin-binding protein and decorin binding proteins A and B. Fibronectin is commonly found in the synovium, and decorin levels are high in the joints. The spirochetes often congregate in the synovia, the viscid lubricating fluid surrounding joints and tendon sheaths. (The spirochetes are also strongly attracted to collagen tissues through other mechanisms than the utilization of decorin or other proteoglycans.)

Lyme spirochetes avidly bind to collagen lattices, grow, and form microcolonies. At binding, they release a unique compound, Oms28—a porin. Porins are usually made and released by lymphocytes and other immune cells. The porins form pores in the outer membranes of cells, hence their name. (These same porins are released wherever Lyme spirochetes travel; they help the organisms penetrate and break down tissues.)

In an attempt to deal with the infection, the immune system stimulates the proliferation of mononuclear cells in the synovial tissue (macrophages, T cells, B cells, and plasma cells). In the joint fluid neutrophils (primarily) as well as immune complexes, complement compounds, and inflammatory cytokines are stimulated. Once this process begins the spirochetes take an active part, stimulating the body's release of a number of unique compounds called matrix metalloproteinases (MMPs). These compounds facilitate the penetration of the spirochetes through extracellular matrix component barriers. The type of MMPs that the spirochetes stimulate differs depending on a number of factors that have not yet been clearly understood. In general, the most common MMPs that are stimulated are MMP-1, -3, and -9. MMP-2, -8, -13, and -19 are also sometimes present. The spirochetes stimulate the monocytes in the synovial fluid to release MMP-1 and the neutrophils in the joint fluid to release MMP-9. MMP-3 is released from chondrocytes (mature cartilage cells) near the articular surface; MMP-1 is also released from primary human chondrocytes. (Lyme spirochetes, in essence, use the human immune system as a tool during infection.)

MMP-1 and MMP-3 production in Lyme arthritis are stimulated through a particular grouping of pathways—mitogen-activated protein kinases (MAPKs), specifically c-Jun N-terminal kinase (JNK), p38 mitogen-activated protein (p38), and extracellular signal-regulated kinase 1/2 (ERK 1/2).

Factors that are involved with the emergence of the different MMPs are spirochete type, its outer protein variation, and the kind of antibiotic therapy that has been used. The spirochetes utilize the impacts of MMPs to facilitate their movement through and presence in tissues and seemingly are able to modify those impacts depending on how the body deals with the infection.

While many MMPs do show up during Lyme infections, the most frequently found and most damaging to tissues seem to be MMP-1, -3, and -9. No Lyme arthritis condition has occurred where one of these three was not strongly present.

The MMPs are strongly implicated in the damage to the joints. However, joint damage does not occur unless plasminogen is also present. Unsurprisingly, Lyme spirochetes possess a plasminogen-binding factor on their outer membrane. In consequence, plasminogen binds to their outer protein coats causing plasminogen concentration increases wherever spirochetes are located. The addition of plasminogen to MMP concentrations results in significant glycosaminoglycan (GAG) and hydroxyproline release and subsequent cartilage damage. As this process proceeds, the spirochetes eventually release a unique protein Bgp— *Borrelia* glycosaminoglycan binding protein—which stimulates binding of GAGs to the spirochetes protein surfaces. GAGs are one of the sources of nutrients for the spirochetes from which they extract sugars.

Inhibition of MMP production has been found to stop GAG releases, prevent cartilage degradation, and inhibit the progression of Lyme arthritis (see *Polygonum cuspidatum*).

Borrelia spirochetes also stimulate the production of Interleukin-16 (IL-16), cyclooxygenase 2 (COX-2), and tumor necrosis factor alpha (TNF-a). They inhibit the production of tissue inhibitor of metalloproteinases (TIMP-1). Levels of CD4+, CD25+, and CD57+ T cells are lower and CD8+ levels are higher during Lyme spirochete infection. (Increases in the levels of either CD8 or TNF-a in the human body also increases levels of IL-16.) Stimulating CD4 and CD25 production (that is, increasing their levels in the body) and balancing the CD4/CD8 ratio have been shown to prevent destructive arthritis during Lyme borreliosis. Anti-interleukin-17 therapy has also been found effective in significantly reducing Lyme arthritis *in vivo*. Modifying the Th1/Th2 balance can also be of help in the treatment of Lyme arthritis. Increasing the production of Th2 components—IL-6 and IL-10—have been shown *in vivo* to reduce the severity of the arthritis.

A great many studies, *in vitro, in vivo,* and in people, have found that the primary factor leading to arthritic inflammations is the health of the immune system. Spirochete levels have been found to be irrelevant to the severity of the disease.

Studies on Lyme arthritis commonly assert that anywhere from 50-80% of "untreated" patients will develop Lyme arthritis and at least 10% will develop antibiotic-resistant Lyme arthritis. "Untreated" means someone who does not immediately receive antibiotics at the onset of Lyme infection. The median onset for Lyme arthritis is approximately four months after infection. Since the telltale EM rash only occurs in about 37% of people, and since new infection rates in the United States are more realistically running from 90,000 to 200,000 people yearly, somewhere between 60,000 and 130,000 people a year are not receiving antibiotics at onset of infection. Lyme arthritis will occur in the U.S. population in anywhere from 30,000 to 104,000 people. Of these somewhere between 3,000 and 10,000 per year are developing antibiotic-resistant Lyme arthritis.

In general, spirochete levels are low during Lyme disease and this is also true of Lyme arthritis. Even with biopsy, spirochetes are difficult to find during active Lyme arthritis. Treatment with antibiotics is helpful to many but still, a significant number continue to present symptoms even with multiple and long-term antibiotic regimens. Even in people who test negative for the disease or in those who have undergone as much as five months of antibiotic therapy, spirochetes have still been found in synovial tissues (even if the synovial fluid is clear). Spirochetal antigens tend to be present as well, in the perivascular areas, in deep synovial stroma among collagen bundles, in vacuoles of fibroblasts in synovial membranes, and in cytophagosomes of mononuclear cells of the synovial fluid. The synovial lining is often thickened and vascular injury is common. (See sections on "Immune Evasion" and "Treatment Failures" this chapter.)

In general, Lyme arthritis usually resolves on its own, even if untreated. Average time for resolution is four years from date of infection, though much longer arthritic complications have been shown to occur. Lyme arthritis is exceptionally responsive to plant-based therapies—see *Polygonum cuspidatum* in chapter three and relevant sections (e.g. stephania root) in chapter four.

Neuroborreliosis:
Lyme Infection of the Central Nervous System

Of the four common areas of symptomatic Lyme infection—skin, joints, heart, and the central nervous system—the latter is often the most debilitating. Onset can be late or immediate and can range from mild to severe. Both central and peripheral nervous systems are frequently involved.

Lyme spirochetes actively invade the cerebral spinal fluid (CSF), the meninges, and the brain shortly after infection. Studies on the rate of spread vary, from 12 hours in mice to one month in rhesus macaques (monkeys). Generally, it is accepted that the spirochetes are established in the central nervous system within 7-14 days, often before the EM rash has time to appear.

The severity of the symptoms that occur from central-nervous-system infection with Lyme spirochetes depends most strongly on the health of the individual's immune system. The type of borrelia spirochete also plays a role as does the length of infection prior to treatment. The longer the spirochetes are in the body prior to treatment, the more adjusted they become to the specific immune situation in that host and the more antigenic variation they will already have created in their offspring. Several studies have found that treatment beyond seven days after infection shows more relapse and more bacterial resistance to treatment than treatment within that first week.

Central nervous system (CNS) complications in neuroborreliosis generally involve inflammatory processes initiated by spirochete invasion of the CNS. This usually includes: meningismus (less common in Europe), lymphocytic meningitis, meningoencephalomyelitis, and subacute encephalopathies. Peripheral nervous system (PNS) involvements are usually inflammation initiated as well: cranial neuropathy, painful radiculitis, sudden sensorineural healing loss, vertigo, vision abnormalities, distal neuropathy, myositis, and polymyalgia rheumatica. Personality changes, mood swings, sleep disorder, cognitive problems, and psychiatric symptoms are common. Chronic borreliosis with primary PNS involvement has been found to average 16 months after infection, with primary CNS aspects in about 26 months. However, many CNS and PNS effects (e.g. cognitive disturbance, memory problems, meningismus) begin to occur within seven days of infection.

There are three membranes that surround and protect the brain and spinal cord, collectively called the meninges. The pia mater adheres to the brain and spinal cord, the dura mater adheres to the bone, and the arachnoid lies between them. Meningitis refers to the inflammation of any or all of these membranes. Meninges involvement is very common in Lyme borreliosis.

Meningismus basically means a stiff neck. It is often accompanied by headaches. Active inflammation may not be found during examination and the cerebral spinal fluid (CSF) may appear normal.

Lymphocytic meningitis occurs from dense collections of lymphocytes (white blood cells) in the meninges. Sometimes the inflammation extends further, into the brain. It is often difficult to distinguish from other forms of meningitis. Headaches, fluctuating in intensity, are common. Up to one third of those infected may experience cranial neuropathy (temporary nerve damage in the face or head). Low-grade encephalopathy is often present in up to one half. More seriously, meningoencephalomyelitis (inflammation of the nerves, meninges, and brain accompanied by focal parenchymal lesions) may sometimes occur.

The most common neuroborreliosis symptom is subacute encephalopathy with attendant memory problems and depression. Sleepiness in the daytime and wakefulness at night are common. Extreme irritability, fatigue, headaches, disorganization, and continual mild incoherence are common. Nerve pain is often present. There are measurable deficits in memory, new learning, retrieval of information, attention and concentration, perceptual-motor skills, and problem solving. In spite of most people's strenuous efforts to overcome these deficits, they are generally unsuccessful in doing so; the spirochete infection of the CNS has too many impacts on cognition. Children tend to have significantly fewer cognitive problems (e.g. memory and thinking) than adults. In adults, the inability to think and solve problems can be severe. It is not uncommon for a person to be walking in front of their house and to not realize that this is where they live. This incapacity has to be taken into account when treating people who have Lyme infections; they may not be able to follow a treatment regimen without help. Numbness or tingling in the extremities, "crawling" sensations, facial weakness, and radiating nerve pain are also very common.

In about 11% of Lyme infections, more often children, a partial facial paralysis (Bell's palsy) occurs. Two thirds of these only affect one side of the face.

While there are a number of conditions that can present similarly to neuroborreliosis, the combination of subacute encephalopathy, peripheral neuropathy, and a Lyme-type arthritis are highly indicative of Lyme infection, specifically neuroborreliosis.

The gaps in our understanding of CNS Lyme disease stem from several factors. First, we lack a definitive assay to demonstrate active infection. Second, Bb infection can be occult, resulting in long periods of latency before symptoms are manifest. Third, Bb can disseminate to sequestered compartments where antibiotic penetration is difficult and immune surveillance is lacking. Fourth, Bb is known to have considerable strain heterogeneity. This strain heterogeneity may result in different levels of virulence and different organotropism... Fifth, the antigenic variability of Bb is known to result in different antigen expression in different locales [in the body]... Sixth, the significance of coinfection with other tick-borne organisms ... is not fully understood... Finally, although there are well-characterized neurologic syndromes associated with early and late stage infection, the full spectrum of neurologic Lyme disease has not yet been fully described.

—Brian Fallon, M.D.
The 12th International Conference on Lyme Disease and Other Spirochetal and Tick-Borne Diseases

Physiological Changes During Neuroborreliosis

The spirochetes tend to invade and cluster within the subarachnoid space in the meninges. (This causes the headache and stiff neck that often accompany infection.) This space is located between the pia mater, or innermost meningeal layer which covers the brain and spinal cord, and the arachnoid layer in the middle of the three meninges. Cerebral spinal fluid (CSF) circulates between the meningeal layers. Just as the spirochetes have an affinity for cartilage in the larger joints of the body, they have an equally strong affinity (tropism) for the meninges. (These two layers are also sometimes called the leptomeninges.)

The leptomeninges, nerve roots, and dorsal root ganglia are where the spirochetes cluster most strongly. In the peripheral nervous system, they localize to the endoneurium and the connective tissues of peripheral nerves.

One of the reasons why Bell's palsy occurs so often with Lyme infections is that when people, usually children, are bitten on the neck (generally near the hairline) the spirochetes are injected close to the site of the long facial nerve. The spirochetes move quickly to the connective tissue in this nerve, causing inflammation that swells the nerve and it seizes up. Borrelia infiltrates cluster near the endoneural vessels of the facial nerve. Peri, epi, and endoneural infiltrations of macrophages, plasma cells, and B cells cause an inflammation of the facial and trigeminal nerves near the site of infection.

In the CNS, the third meningeal layer—the dura mater—which adheres to the bone, may sometimes be colonized as well. Spirochete-stimulated inflammation in the meninges can be mild or severe. The weaker the immune system, the more inflammation usually occurs. Later stages often show more inflammation as the spirochetes have adapted more effectively to the host immune response.

Upon the establishment of the spirochetes in the meninges, white blood cells, primarily lymphocytes, emerge in the cerebral spinal fluid (pleocytosis) to fight the infection. A host of other immune complexes are upregulated. As brain macrophages (microglia) attempt to deal with the infection by upregulating their production, tumor necrosis factor-alpha (TNF alpha), Interleukin-1 alpha, interferon-gamma

(IFN-gamma), prostaglandin E2 (PGE2), and interleukin-6 levels increase substantially. IL-4 levels, in contrast, are exceptionally low in those with chronic neuroborreliosis (NB) while in early NB infection, IL-4 levels are higher. (The upregulation of IFN-gamma persists in the brain up to four months after the end of treatment with antibiotics.) Nuclear factor-kappa B (NF-kB) is induced and increased expression of Toll-like receptor 2 and CD14 also occur.

Lymphocyte levels of CD4+, CD8+, HLA-DR+, and total T lymphocytes, B lymphocytes, and NK cells are all high. CD8+ production is especially high and expresses in turn C-C chemokine receptor 5 and CD69. Chemokines, a unique form of cytokine with strong chemotactic actions, are elevated. Interleukin-8 (IL-8) and macrophage inflammatory protein 1 alpha and 1 beta (MIP-1a, MIP-1b) levels all elevate— MIP-1b and IL-8 significantly so. After antibiotic treatment, IL-8, MIP-1a, and -1b levels decline but generally not to preinfectious levels.

The spirochetes that occur in the CNS are antigenetically very different than those that infect the rest of the body. Those in the CNS tend to be neurotrophic, that is, attracted to neural cells. Once they colonize the meninges they can penetrate brain tissue. Normally this happens late in the infection or when the immune system is depressed. Direct spinal-cord involvement is rare though it can happen, generally in the severely immunocompromised. Levels of IgG, IgM, and Clq in the cord are high. (Clq is a protein activated by the complement system. It increases vascular permeability, attraction of polymorphonuclear leukocytes, enhances phagocytosis, and alters cell membrane structures.)

After the spirochetes are well established in the meninges, they will often begin to penetrate the brain, adhering to the brain's glial cells, especially the neuroglia, astrocytes, and microglia. The neuroglia is a supporting tissue that is intermingled with other tissues throughout the brain. Microglia are scattered throughout the brain and central nervous system and essentially act like macrophages. That is, upon infection, they are activated to fight it. (See section on Lyme Neurotoxins, this chapter.) Astrocytes are brain cells that are also capable of phagocytosis. They are fairly large, star-shaped (hence their name—*astro* means star), and support the nerve cells (neurons) of the brain and spinal cord.

Basically, spirochetes adhere to both nerve roots and brain cells, causing changes in both.

Different types of proteoglycans contribute to the spirochetes' ability to bind to brain cells. Binding is inhibited by substances that interfere with proteoglycan synthesis and by exogenous (externally supplied) proteoglycans, e.g. heparin. (That is why heparin taken along with antibiotics has been found to help cure the disease.) Perivascular or vasculitic lymphocytic inflammation may occur. Hypoperfusion (decreased blood flow) of the frontal subcortical and cortical structures is common. This will partially reverse upon antibiotic therapy but has been found to be present, though at much lower levels, in those with post-lyme-disease syndrome and those who have been treated successfully with antibiotics. Cerebral atrophy is common, and in a small percentage of cases both the white matter and brain stem can sustain damage. Demyelination of the nerves where the spirochetes cluster and in the periventricular white matter can occur as well. Demyelination means that the myelin sheaths that surround and protect the nerves are degraded. This slows down the nerve impulse tranmission considerably. Demyelination is a primary problem in multiple sclerosis (MS) which is why many neuroborreliosis and MS symptoms are, in some instances, so similar.

As an aside, recent research has found that in a number of Alzheimer's patients, at autopsy, particular kinds of dental treponema spirochetes were present in the brain. They infected the brain via branches of the trigeminal nerve. (See Riviere, et al. "Molecular and immunological evidence of oral Treponema in the human brain and their association with Alzheimer's disease," *Oral Microbiol Immunol* 2002 Apr;17(2):113-8.) Another study found Lyme spirochetes in the brain of three Alzheimer's patients at autopsy. The organisms were identified as *Borrelia burgdorferi sensu stricto*. Borrelia antigens and genes were co-localized with beta-amyloid deposits in the brain. The patients had been correctly diagnosed with Alzheimer's disease and the brain damage was consistent with that diagnosis. (See Miklossy, et al. "Borrelia burgdorferi persists in the brain in chronic Lyme neuroborreliosis and may be associated with Alzheimer's disease." *Journal of*

Alzheimer's Disease, 2004;6(6):no page numbers available.) Spirochete presence—not necessarily *Borrelia*—in the brain may also be a factor for those with multiple sclerosis. Lida Mattman, a professor at the Department of Biology at Wayne State University and a Nobel nominee for her work on stealth pathogens has apparently identified spirochetes as the causative agent in multiple sclerosis. This could explain both the evolution of the disease and why bee venom injections have been found to be of help. Melittin, the primary component in bee venom is particularly effective against spirochetes.

As with Lyme arthritis, spirochetes in the CNS cause the upregulation of metalloproteinases. The production of MMP-9 and 130 kDa gelatinase (aka MMP130) are strongly stimulated in affected cells such as astrocytes. MMP-3 has also been found in the spinal fluid of those with neuroborreliosis. MMPs can break down extracellular matrix glycoproteins and proteoglycans (components of cartilage) as well as the myelin sheaths that surround the nerves.

Spirochete numbers in the CNS are often low and, again, they tend to alter their form considerably. Significant antigenic variation is common and the spirochetes in the nervous system can differ from those in the rest of the body considerably. Those in the CNS often downregulate OspC proteins and upregulate OspA. So CNS spirochetes can be OspA dominant while spirochetes in other locations may be OspC dominant. The different antigenic nature of the spirochetes (individually and throughout the world) produce different impacts. In Europe, CNS infection has been found to be accompanied by prominent CSF abnormalities, while in the U.S. the spinal fluid often appears normal (except in late-stage neuroborreliosis where one third of those infected will show abnormal readings). In numerous studies, intentionally infected animals will produce types of spirochetes in the CNS that do not exist in the laboratory ticks that infected them.

Spirochetes in the CNS also tend to encyst rather than remain in their elongated form (see section on Immune Evasion). These cysts, if removed and placed in growth medium, will reconvert to spirochetal form. This is one of the reasons that spirochetes are often not detected in spinal fluid.

Post Lyme Disease Syndrome

A great many people who have had Lyme disease or lengthy CNS infections with the Lyme spirochetes, report continual problems even after apparently successful antibiotic treatment. I will deal with some of this later (See Treatment Failures and Immune Evasion). However, there has been a considerable amount of research on the long-term impacts of borrelial infection in the CNS.

These data demonstrate that Lyme neuroborreliosis is a persistent infection, that spirochetal presence is a necessary but not sufficient condition for inflammation, and that antibody measured in serum may not predict the severity of infection.

—AR PACHNER, et al. "Central and Nervous System infection, immunity, and inflammation in the NHP model of Lyme borreliosis"

As mentioned earlier, hypoperfusion in the brain in many instances does not completely reverse after antibiotic treatment. IL-8, MIP-1a and -1b levels generally do decline but not to preinfectious levels, and levels of IFN-gamma can remain high for months after antibiotic regimens are completed. The demyelinization of the nerves can produce long term problems. There are, in a number of cases, persistent spirochetal infections of the CNS that do not respond to treatment. Although a bit dated given the rapidity of Lyme research findings, the best look at this is the special issue of *Applied Neuropsychology* which focused entirely on the "Neuropsychological Aspects of Lyme Disease" (Kaplan, editor, 1999; 6(1)). In short, repeated and very sophisticated testing of antibiotic-treated NB patients found that they did in fact show cognitive problems that were outside the norm, though not as severe as those with active neuroborreliosis.

The white-matter regions of the brain where the most hypoperfusion occurs during Lyme disease are part of the large-scale, neurocognitive networks that are involved in mediating memory and attention. Additionally, it has been found that during Lyme infection alterations in hippocampal function occurs as well. The hippocampus is intimately concerned with memory and memory retrieval. More than 50% of

those with late-stage NB, even if treated, experience subjective symptoms of memory-retrieval impairment, working-memory dysfunction,
and impaired attention. More than one-third experience depression or
anxiety and report continuing sleep problems. Tests show that there are
impairments in measures of memory, verbal fluency, attention, and
dexterity compared to controls. In other words, while it may be in their
heads, they are not making it up.

These results show that for many, antibiotic treatment alone is
insufficient. With the caveat that some post-Lyme-disease syndrome
patients are experiencing immune evasion by the spirochete and an
unrecognized treatment failure, the studies indicate that additional supportive protocols are necessary to help correct brain impacts from the
infection. While pharmaceuticals are inept for this purpose, plants are
not, and in many instances have been found specific for the problems
that occur in post-Lyme-disease syndrome.

Quinolinic Acid: A Potent Neurotoxin in Neuroborreliosis

In addition to the direct damage that occurs in the central nervous system during neuroborreliosis, a central nervous system toxin, quinolinic
acid, is also produced and has potent impacts on brain function.

Microglia, derived from stem cells during embryo development, are considered to be the primary macrophages of the brain. They normally constitute about 4% of brain tissue and are generally inactive. But when microbial infection in the brain does occur the microglia become highly activated. Once activated these cells prolifer-ate and can represent a significant volume of brain tissue. They then

Quinolinic acid accumulation in brain tissue contributes to atrophy in vulnerable brain regions.

—MELVYN HAYES, et al.
"Elevated Cerebrospinal fluid quinolinic acid levels are associated with cerebral volume loss in HIV infection"

produce large quantities of quinolinic acid (QUIN). The amount of
QUIN can be very high in the CSF and the brain—much higher than
blood tests are able to show. High levels of QUIN have been found in

neuro-degenerative diseases such as Parkinson's, Alzheimer's, Huntington's, and AIDS dementia.

In chronic neuroborreliosis, QUIN levels in the CSF are consistently
elevated (35 nmols), while during acute episodes these levels can
increase nearly ten times (325 nmols). Levels in the brain are substantially higher than those in the CSF. Tests of the impact of QUIN on the
brain have found that levels from 40 to 80 nmols produce little neuronal
loss in the hippocampus while 120 nmols can produce over 90% neuronal loss. However, when QUIN levels increase in the presence of reactive oxygen species (ROS), the ROS significantly potentiate the effects of
QUIN. The addition of ROS to QUIN causes 80% neuronal loss in the
hippocampus at 80 nmols. The levels of QUIN generally found in acute
neuroborreliosis approach the low end of those found in neurological
AIDS infections and AIDS dementia.

Macrophages and polymorphonuclear leukocytes, human immune
cells, routinely produce reactive oxygen species (ROS) during bacterial
infections. ROS are potent bacteriocidal agents and are created to kill
Lyme spirochetes. Lyme spirochetes have been found to be exceptionally
potent stimulators of ROS production, more so than other spirochetes
such as those that cause syphilis and leptospira. Additionally, *Borrelia
burgdorferi sensu lato* are exceptionally sensitive to alterations in oxygen
levels during infection, and they actively begin to alter their gene
expression and antigenic profiles to escape its effects. They do this
through a specific transcriptional activator—the *Borrelia* oxidative
stress response regulator or BosR.

When Lyme spirochetes invade the CNS and brain they cause a
potent stimulation of QUIN by macrophages AND significant ROS production. These two substances act synergistically to damage the CNS. In
many respects, QUIN is considered a *pro*-oxidant rather than an antioxidant. It potentiates the effects of free-radicals and other reactive oxygen
species on tissues, especially the brain. QUIN also induces the production of nuclear factor-kappa B (NF-kB). NFkB also acts as an neurotoxin, exacerbating neuronal death.

QUIN impact on the brain and brain function has been found to be severe. This includes such things as neurotransmitter interference, damage to the synaptic connections, brain atrophy, cerebral volume loss, and neuronal death. Major areas of impact are the hippocampus, the striatum, limbic cortex, neocortex, and amygdala. The main problems associated with these are memory and recall deficits and confusion. The impairment of performance on memory-related tasks found in CNS Lyme infection and PLDS is consistent with elevated QUIN levels. Without specific therapies designed to protect the brain from QUIN impacts and to stimulate regeneration of damaged areas, the damage is unlikely to correct. Antibiotics alone can do nothing to either protect or help regenerate areas susceptible to the neurotoxic effects of QUIN. (See "Neuroborreliosis' in chapter four.)

Additionally, QUIN levels tend to be exacerbated in older people, a natural aspect of aging. This correlates with the more severe impacts of neuroborreliosis in older people and the tendency among them for long-term problems in memory and other cognitive functions.

Lyme Carditis

Heart complications occur in about 10% of those with Lyme infections. This commonly shows as rhythm or conduction abnormalities, endomyocarditis, or pericarditis. Partial atrioventricular block (an electrical conduction problem) is the most common problem. Occasionally, total block does occur which is much more dangerous. The three main symptoms are chest pain, heart palpitations, and shortness of breath.

There are three primary physiological locations for the spirochete during Lyme carditis. Early in the infection they locate in and around the blood vessels (in the lumen or perivascular space) surrounding the heart. As the disease progresses the spirochetes invade cardiac monocytes. Finally, they cluster to the collagen fibers, wrapping around the fibers with their long axis parallel to the fibers themselves. Inflammatory infiltrates invade the pericardium and endocardium. Spirochete numbers, as with other sites in the body, tend to be low, out of proportion to the severity of the disease.

Ocularborreliosis and Otoborreliosis

Lyme infection does cause regular eye problems, though this is often overlooked. The most common problems are "floaters," feeling of pressure in the eyes, and disturbed vision. Optic nerve disease, neuroretinitis, conjunctivitis, keratitis, uveitis, vitreitis, and other forms of posterior segment inflammatory disease do occur, especially in highly endemic areas. Chronic and acute anterior uveitis is probably the most common complication. This is an inflammation of the frontal membranes of the iris and choroid. Pain and redness are the main symptoms. Spirochetes have been isolated from iris tissues but they mainly tend to locate in the aqueous humor. They have been isolated from tears. All this is very similar to the meninges/brain relationship in Lyme infections. Normally, the spirochetes limit themselves to the membranes and the fluid but occasionally will penetrate deeper into the underlying tissues, which is when more severe pathology occurs.

Ear complications are common as well. The primary problems are buzzing or ringing in the ears, sound sensitivity, motion sickness, vertigo, and poor balance. Sudden sensorineural hearing loss (SHL) can occur as well. Neurological Lyme infection tends to affect the cochlear part of the nerve of the ear, though the vestibular section can also be affected. Serological evidence of Lyme infection has been reported in one-fifth of people affected by SHL. Vertigo is present in somewhere between 8%-30% of people with Lyme borreliosis. Buzzing or ringing in the ears (tinnitus) and vertigo are probably the most common problems.

Immune Evasion

The Lyme spirochetes, as mentioned earlier, can change their outer membrane structure quickly and often. Spirochetes that do not express OspC generally survive in hosts that develop an anti-OspC antibody response. However, if those non-OspC spirochetes are taken and injected into mice that do not have an anti-OspC antibody production, the spirochetes will begin recombining to include OspC forms.

As the immune system recognizes that an infection is occurring, it begins targeting the spirochetes themselves. As soon as this occurs, the spirochetes begin altering their forms to evade the immune response.

For example, in response to immune attack, OspC expression decreases by 446 times. BBFO1 and VslE (two other surface proteins on the spirochetes outer membrane) increase up to 20 and 32 times respectively.

Spirochetes that strongly bind to decorin are much better protected than those that do not. Decorin expression is higher in joints and skin than in the urinary bladder and heart, and spirochetes that express an outer protein coat high in decorin-binding proteins survive much better than those that do not. For example, spirochetes that congregate in the synovial fluid—the viscid lubricating fluid surrounding joints and tendon sheaths—are exceptionally difficult to eradicate. Treatment with antibiotics will kill the spirochetes that exist loosely in the fluid. It turns out, however, that the spirochetes also enter into the synovial cells themselves where they are protected from both immune attack and antibiotics. After the assault ends, the spirochetes exit the cells and spread once more through the body. The Lyme spirochetes that actively invade host cells can be detected alive inside them surrounded by a shielding membrane that they have constructed. This intracellular sequestering occurs with a number of different kinds of cells—synovial, macrophages, fibroblasts, and endothelial. This allows the spirochetes to evade the immune response and antibacterial agents and engage in long-term persistent infections.

Any assault, whether from the immune system or from antibiotics, causes Lyme spirochetes to immediately initiate evasion tactics. In addition to the kinds of alterations discussed above, the spirochetes can do more—they can take on or create completely different spirochetal forms. These are generally referred to as cysts (or encysted forms), blebs, and spheroblast L-forms. During their growth phase, Lyme spirochetes shed copious quantities of what are referred to as blebs. These are granules of DNA plasmids, both circular and linear. Among other things the blebs appear to act as congregants for IgM antibodies. Blebs may bind all or most of the circulating IgM, helping the spirochetes to evade immune detection. In essence, this is much like a plane releasing a spray of metal fragments in order to confuse radar readings.

These spirochete blebs are also taken up by different human cells—dendritic cells, lymphocytes, and fibroblasts—where they move into the cytosol and nucleus of the cells. Why this happens is unknown but CD8(+) cells actively attack those cells that have taken in the blebs and kill them. Speculation (again) has been that this might be an aspect of the autoimmune aspects of Lyme borreliosis. To date, the real purposes of bleb shedding are unknown.

Antibiotic regimens can cause the alteration of spirochetes into abnormal motile forms—spheroblast L-forms as well as encysted forms. Antibody production, high heat (as in fever), and extreme pH alterations can also stimulate encysted-form development. When Lyme spirochetes move into the cerebral spinal fluid (CSF), all spirochetes encyst with 24 hours, leaving no motile forms. Additionally, when spirochetes are starved, they immediately encyst. Ninety-five percent of the spirochetes that are starved can encyst within one minute. If these encysted forms are then placed in a medium rich in food, they will convert once again to motile spirochetes within 9-17 days. (The older the cysts are the fewer that will reconvert to motile forms.) Every part of the body that the spirochetes invade have also been found to contain encysted forms of the organism, irrespective of starvation, antibiotics, or immune response. The capacity of spirochetes such as Lyme organisms to encyst has been recognized since 1905, but the information was ignored until recently when repeated infections began occurring in people who had received antibiotic regimens.

These altered forms of the spirochete, though incompletely understood, are sophisticated mechanisms for ensuring persistence of the organism in multiple environments and in the face of strenuous immune assault. The end effect of the spirochete being able to persist intracellularly, to shed blebs, to take on alternate motile forms, to encyst, and to emerge from an encysted form when conditions are more favorable is persistent infection in spite of human-immune response and antibiotic treatment.

Immune Dynamics in Chronic Lyme

A number of studies have found that a subset of the body's natural killer cells (NK) becomes severely depressed in chronic or late-stage Lyme infections. This subset, denoted CD57+, is an aggressive white blood cell or lymphocyte that seems to be specific for Lyme spirochetes. Lyme borrelia, it now appears, can disable these NK cells. People with low CD57 levels have been found to have more coinfections, more neurological symptoms, and persistent immunological defects compared to those with higher CD57 levels. People with Lyme that will not resolve, even with multiple courses of antibiotics, have been found to have low CD57 levels; this appears to be a reliable diagnostic marker for unresolved Lyme. (See for example, Stricker, et al. Long-term decrease in the CD57 lymphocyte subset in a patient with chronic Lyme disease. *Ann Agric Environ Med* 2002, 9:111-113.) CD57 counts are apparently normal in early stage Lyme infections; they begin to be reduced after the organism has established itself and adapted to the particular host ecology. A test for CD57 levels exists and can be used to track the course of successful treatment (see the resource section at rear of book and cat's claw [*Uncaria tomentosa*] in chapter three for more).

Herxheimer Reactions

Herxheimer reactions or Herxing (aka Jarisch-Herxheimer reaction) is named after early bacterial researchers, Adolph Jarisch and Karl Herxheimer, who first described the condition. It occurs during a large die-off of bacterial organisms in the progress of a disease or its treatment. Herxheimer reactions are common in Lyme infections. When antibiotics are given and large numbers of spirochetes die, their bodies fragment. These body parts and associated toxins that they release cause a temporary worsening of symptoms. It is a good indication of the effectiveness of a medication in the early stages of treatment. These reactions can be ameliorated by the use of substances that bind endotoxins or lessened by lowering the dose of the drug or herb being used. (Endotoxins, in this instance, means substances released by bacteria when they die. These can often make people feel more ill than when the bacteria are alive and healthy. See "Herxheimer Reactions" in chapter four.)

Treatment Failures with Lyme Borreliosis

☞

The optimal treatment of various forms of LB is unknown. Most
of the therapeutic trials have drawbacks if evaluated critically,
and their results have to be interpreted with caution.
— MIIKKA PELTOMAA, University of Helsinki, 1999.

In the antibiotic treatment of Lyme infections, the primary oral antibiotics used are amoxicillin, doxycycline, cefuroxime axetil, clar-
ithromycin, and metronidazole. The primary parenteral antibiotics are
ceftriaxone, cefotaxime, doxycycline, azithromycin, vancomycin,
unisyn, and ampicillin IV.

The standard treatment duration for Lyme infection in the United
States is considered to be 10-28 days. While this does work for some,
there is significant evidence that perhaps for 40% of people who are
infected it does not. Studies routinely show that up to 95% of people are
"cured" by antibiotics with this duration of treatment. Often neglected
in this discussion is that there are 5% who are not. Additionally, there is
commonly up to a 35% relapse rate that necessitates repeated antibiotic
therapies. Some studies have found that a longer initial treatment regimen reduces or eliminates relapse.

A great many studies have shown that there is a significant population of people, treated with the accepted regimen of antibiotics, who do
not get well and who still have spirochete loads in their bodies. For
many of them, the long duration of infection due to improper antibiotic dosing significantly worsens their conditions.

Conflicts between physicians who feel that short antibiotic regimens are sufficient and those who have found in practice that they are
not, are severe. Regrettably, the conflict cannot be, though it should be,
resolved by a reliance on the data and the experience of individual
physicians. The primary reason for the lack of attention to the clinical
data appears to be financial. Insurance companies do not want years-
long antibiotic therapy to become an accepted protocol because of the
effect on their bottom lines. (The scatological nature of that obsession

seemingly escapes them.) This same kind of controversy occurred during the early years of the AIDS epidemic.

As Harry Goldhagen and Julie Rawlings comment in their article "Lyme Disease Controversies:"

> *But why be concerned [about longer uses of antibiotics]? Guidelines are not ironclad rules for treatment. Physicians generally individualize treatment, using their clinical judgement when a presentation varies from the typical or when the patient doesn't respond to first-line treatment. Individualization is the basis of medical care.*
>
> *If only that were still true. In the United States, most medical care is paid for by insurance companies—managed care organizations, preferred provider organizations, and other healthcare companies. Insurance companies use guidelines from respected medical groups to determine whether treatments should be "covered" and which should not. Therefore, if a set of guidelines suggests that there is no evidence to support certain types of treatment, it can be difficult or impossible for the patient and physician to receive reimbursement from the insurance company.*

Worse still, is that many physicians who have used longer-term antibiotic therapies have found themselves brought before their respective medical boards in the U.S., and threatened with loss of license if they did not stop the longer antibiotic protocols. This is especially reprehensible given that there is a large body of clinical evidence that supports longer therapies for many people. There have been serious impacts on physicians and people who have Lyme and there is no clear explanation for it except this: that it interferes with the profit margins of powerful corporations.

The data on antibiotic failures are clear. What follows is only a brief review. All are direct quotes from the research papers themselves.

- *If treatment with vancomycin was delayed for 7 days or more [after infection], vancomycin failed to eradicate infection with B. burgdorferi of B. turicatae from immunodeficient mice. The failure of vancomycin in eradicating established infections in immunodeficient mice was associated with the persistence of viable spirochetes in the brain during antibiotic treatment.* (Kazragis, et al. In vivo activities of ceftriaxone and vancomycin against Borrelia spp. in the mouse brain, and other sites. *Antimicrob Agents Chemother,* 1996 Nov;40(11)2632-6.)

- *Despite antibiotic therapy, there was progression to a chronic stage, with multisystem manifestations. The initially significant immune system activation was followed by a loss of the specific humoral immune response and a decrease in the cellular immune response to B. burgdorferi over the course of the disease. "Trigger finger" developed, and a portion of the flexor retinaculum obtained at surgery was cultured. Viable spirochetes were identified. Ultramorphologically, the spirochetes were situated between collagen fibers and along fibroblasts, some of which were deeply invaginated by these organisms.* (T. Haupl, et al. "Persistence of Borrelia burgdorferi in ligamentous tissue from a patient with chronic Lyme borreliosis." Arthritis and Rheumatism 1993;36(11):1621-1626.)

- *A total of 165 patients with disseminated Lyme borreliosis (diagnosed in 1990-94, all seropositive except one culture-positive patient) were followed after antibiotic treatment, and 32 of them were regarded as having a clinically defined treatment failure.* (Oksi, et al. "Borrelia burgdorferi detected by culture and PCR in clinical relapse of disseminated Lyme borreliosis" *Ann Med* 1999 Jun;31(3):225-32.)

- *24 volunteers from Connecticut (11 male and 13 female, 7 to 69 years of age [mean, 48.2]) with clinically diagnosed Lyme disease, all of whom had received antibiotic treatment, and 24 healthy volunteers (12 male and 12 female, 23-53 years of age [mean, 35.7]) from Australia, where Lyme disease is not endemic, were recruited into the study… With this criterion [of testing for Lyme disease], 16 (67%) of 24 Lyme patients treated for Lyme disease had a positive test result, while 23 (96%) of 24 control subjects were negative.* (Sikand, et al, "Diagnosis of Lyme borreliosis by a whole-blood gamma interferon assay for cell-mediated immune responses," *Clinical and Diagnostic Laboratory Immunology,* 1999 May; 6(3):445.)

- *102 samples were tested blindly, and 40 samples were retested in a second laboratory. In the first laboratory, B. burgdorferi DNA was detected in CSF samples in 6 (35%) of 16 patients with acute neuroborreliosis, 11(25%) of 44 with chronic neuroborreliosis, and none of 42 samples from patients with other illnesses. There was a significant correlation between PCR results and the duration of previous intravenous antibiotic therapy.* (Nocton, et al. Detection of Borrelia burgdorferi DNA by polymerase chain reaction in cerebrospinal fluid in Lyme neuroborreliosis, *J Infect Dis* 1996 Sept;174(3):623-7.)

- *Eleven patients with neuro-borreliosis had been treated with 200 mg fluconazole daily for 25 days after an unsuccessful therapy with antibiotics. At the end of treatment eight patients had no borreliosis symptoms and remained free of relapse in a follow-up examination one year later. In the remaining four [sic] patients, symptoms were considerably improved.* (Schardt, Clinical effects of fluconazole in patients with neuroborreliosis. *Eur J Res* 2004 Jul 30;9(7):334-6.)

- *A total of 101 patients with acute or chronic neuroborreliosis (proven by clinical data, leukocytosis in the CSF, and elevated Borrelia burgdorferi-specific antibody indices) were treated with 2gm of ceftriaxone per day for either 2 or 3 weeks. The patients were reexamined clinically and serologically after 3, 6, and 12 months. Six (12) months after antibiotic treatment, about 93% (95%) of the patients with acute neuroborreliosis and 20% (66%) of the patients with chronic neuroborreliosis were cured.* (Kaiser, Clinical courses of acute and chronic neuroborreliosis following treatment with ceftriaxone, *Nerevenarzt* 2004 Jun;75(6):553-7.)

- *47 patients with chronic Lyme disease. All had relapsed after long-term oral and intravenous antibiotics. 23 patients with other chronic illnesses formed the control group. Positive cultures were confirmed by fluorescent antibody immuno-electron microscopy using monoclonal antibody directed against OspA, and Osp A PCR. 43/47 patients (91%) cultured positive. 23/23 controls (100%) cultured negative.* (Phillips, et al. A proposal for the reliable culture of

Borrelia burgdorferi from patients with chronic Lyme disease, even from those previously aggressively treated. *Infection* 1998 Nov-Dec;26(6):354-357.)

• *Failures in the antibiotic therapy of Lyme disease have repeatedly been demonstrated by post-treatment isolations of the infecting borreliae.* (Henneberg and Neubert, Borrelia burgdorferi group: in vitro antibiotic sensitivity, *Orv Hetil* 2002 May 26;143(21):1195-8.)

• *35 patients with late stage Lyme borreliosis with involvement of the joints was followed up until 3 years after a 14 day course of 2g ceftriaxone once daily i.v. Diagnosis was confirmed by indirect and direct microbiological methods as well as clinical signs and symptoms. Long term clinical results in 26 patients at 36 months were complete response or marked improvement in 19, relapse in six and new manifestations in four of the cases, respectively.* (Valesova, et al. Long term results in patients with Lyme arthritis following treatment with ceftriaxone. *Infection* 1996 Jan-Feb;24(1):98-102.)

• *Our results show the intra-articular persistence of B. burgdorferi nucleic acids in Lyme arthritis and suggest that persistent organisms and their components are important in maintaining ongoing immune and inflammatory processes even among some antibiotic-treated patients.* (Bradley, et al. The persistence of spirochetal nucleic acids in active Lyme arthritis, *Annals of Internal Medicine*, 1994 March 15;120(6):487-9.)

• *Starting at day 120 after tick challenge, 12 dogs were treated with antibiotics (azithromycin, ceftriaxone, of doxycycline) for 30 consecutive days. Four dogs received no antibiotic therapy... All 16 dogs became infected with B. burgdorferi after tick challenge. In skin biopsy samples, spirochete numbers peaked at day 60 post infection (<1.5x10 to the 6th organisms per 100 ug of extracted DNA), at the same time when clinical signs of arthritis developed in 11 of 16 dogs, and decreased to almost undetectable levels during the following 6 months... Antibiotic treatment reduced the amount of detectable spirochete DNA in skin tissue by a factor of 1,000 or more. At the end* *of the experiment, B. burgdorferi DNA was detectable at low levels (10 squared to 10 to the fourth organisms per ug of extracted DNA) in multiple tissue samples regardless of treatment.* (Straubinger, PCR-based quantification of Borrelia burgdorferi organisms in canine tissues over a 500-day postinfection period, *Journal of Clinical Microbiology*, 2000 June;38(6):2191-9.)

Testing for Lyme Borreliosis

🐚

Despite many of the problems associated with laboratory tests for Lyme disease (sensitivity, specificity, false positives, false negatives, potential cross-reactivity) many physicians rely upon or at least request supplemental information from, serologic tests performed on suspect patient's blood samples.

—DENNIS WHITE, "Lyme Disease Surveillance."

In the absence of a clear-cut erythema migrans rash, there is no way to reliably and consistently diagnose Lyme disease. Up to two thirds of people infected with *Borrelia* have no rash at all and many never see the ticks. The nymph-stage ticks are very small and often missed. While the tests that are used can sometimes help, and while some unusual and not-easily-obtained tests are significantly better, tests consistently miss infection with the spirochetes. A great many people, formerly pronounced seronegative, upon retesting with more sensitive tests or better laboratories have been found to have had Lyme infection all along. There are a number of reasons for the problems with testing.

In the first two-to-four weeks of infection, only about half of infected people produce measurable antibodies to Lyme spirochetes. People tested during this time often test negative and only retest when their health deteriorates significantly. IgM antibodies rise during the third week, peak after 4-6 weeks and then disappear by week eight. IgG antibodies can persist for years or decades after successful treatment and so, when tested, people will be found to be positive for the disease even if they do not have it. Antibody response can be weak or nonexistent at different stages of the disease in different people. Spirochete levels tend to peak at 60 days after infection and then drop to low levels in the system. The spirochete levels may be so low that they do not show and cannot be found even through biopsy. Additionally, they may encyst, making them even more difficult to find. Antibiotic therapies can cause the spirochete levels, already low, to drop by a factor of 1,000 in the body, making detection of any remaining spirochetes nearly impossible by any means. Additionally, false positives, false negatives, cross-reactivity, and other problems are common with the tests for this illness. The primary diagnostic criteria, of necessity, have remained individual and symptomatic with the tests being used as a backup for diagnosis. For an in-depth analysis of the problems with the current testing approaches advocated by the CDC, see the ILADS position paper at www.ilads.org/cdc_paper.html (accessed 2/5/05).

The two most common tests used for Lyme borreliosis are the Elisa and Western Blot. The CDC recommends a two-tiered testing process using these in spite of the fact that the Elisa test is exceptionally unreliable. You and your physician should not rely on it.

Elisa essentially tests blood serum for the presence of antibodies to borrelia organisms. However, it has been found to show negative for at least 35% of those who have had a skin biopsy that included cultivatable spirochetes. There are a significant number of studies that have shown that the test does not work well for this condition. Stanek, et al. commented that "serological results are not supportive for the diagnosis of erythema migrans, nor will they retrospectively prove successful antibiotic treatment of borrelia infection." (Erythema migrans and serodiagnosis by enzyme immunoassay and immunoblot with three borrelia species, *Wien Klin Wochenschr* 1999 Dec 10;111(22-23):951-956). Lomholt, et al. noted that "treatment of erythema migrans should be initiated on clinical appearance as a substantial number of patients stayed seronegative." Their study showed that 41% stayed seronegative with the Elisa test in spite of having a well-developed EM rash and cultivatable spirochetes from the lesion. (Long term serological follow-up of patients treated for chronic cutaneous borreliosis or culture-positive erythema migrans, *Acta Derm Venereol* 2000 Sept-Oct;80(5):362-6.) Other diseases may cause Elisa to show positive as will any past infection with Lyme borreliosis. Everyone who has been vaccinated shows positive with Elisa. These kinds of studies, and there are many more, consistently show that the Elisa test is unreliable. Regrettably, it is still used by physicians due to CDC support of two-tiered testing. The Western Blot is better.

The Western Blot (aka immunoblot) test may be oriented around either IgG or IgM (immunoglobulin G or M), two different antibodies that are produced in response to infection. The test works something like this.

Borrelia spirochetes are killed and broken apart by washing them in a detergent. This separates the proteins from their membranes. A process is then used to bond these proteins to a nylon membrane. Proteins of the same molecular size cluster together and bond to the nylon in what are called "bands." A patient's blood serum is taken and tested with this borrelia-banded nylon sheet to see how many bands the blood reacts with. The more bands the better.

To be usable, the results of Western Blot tests should be reported by showing which bands are reactive. Unfortunately, many labs simply report negative or positive. If you are being tested, you should make sure that the lab reports the bands that react with your blood. The 41kd bands are those that react with the flagella or the motile organs of the spirochete. These are usually the first to react to infection but can cross-react with other spirochetal organisms such as those that cause syphilis. The 18kd, 37kd, 39kd, 83kd, 93kd, 23-25kd (which reflects the presence of OspC), 31kd (which reflects OspA), and 34kd (which reflects OspB) bands are the most specific for Lyme infection. (For some reason the CDC eliminated the use of the 31kd and 34kd bands in the reportable diagnosis of Lyme infection, even though these bands are highly indicative of Lyme exposure.) Bands other than the 41kd typically appear later in the infection and many, sometimes all, may not appear at all. For a positive Lyme test, the 41kd band and at least one of the others have to appear at testing. (Some sources feel that four bands are necessary to make a clinical Lyme diagnosis.) Even if you do have Lyme infection this may not happen. Some 20%-30% of people with Lyme infection may remain seronegative with this test.

Hernandez-Novoa, et al. comment that "In 4.8% of the cases no IgG bands were present and in 26.2% no IgM bands were present" in the Western Blot diagnosis of people with confirmed Lyme infection. (Utility of a commercial immunoblot kit (BAG-Borrelia blot) in the diagnosis of the preliminary stages of Lyme disease, *Diagn Microbiol Infect Dis* 2003 Sep:47(1):321-9.) Bazovska, et al. note that "Lyme borreliosis was clinically established in 19 patients; antibodies to B. burgdorferi were only found in 13 patients in all three tests, and in 4 patients only in the indirect IF test. The results of serological tests for antibodies to B. burgdorferi should be interpreted with caution, as the tests are not standardized and may show false positive or false negative results... The results of serological tests have only supportive value and cannot be deemed conclusive when establishing an etiological diagnosis." (Significance of specific antibody determination in Lyme borreliosis diagnosis, *Bratisl Lek Listy* 2001;102(10):454-7). And Lange and Seyyedi state "the quality of these indirect serological tests and, most importantly, the interpretation criteria of the commercial tests vary dramatically. The choice of Borrelia strains, antigen preparation, production conditions and test procedures vary widely. The immunoblot, used as a confirmatory assay, must meet the highest quality standards but in practice under routine laboratory conditions, these levels are often not reached." (Evidence of a Lyme borreliosis infection from the viewpoint of laboratory medicine, *Int J Med Microbiol* 2002 Jun;291 (Suppl 33):120-4).

Some people are interested in using PCR or polymerase chain reaction in the testing for Lyme disease. This uses the spirochetal DNA itself and enhances it to countable levels. In some instances this is a good test but again its sensitivity is not up to the job in this particular condition. The major problem is that the spirochetes are often in very low numbers and are not homogenous in tissues so that DNA cannot, in many instances be found. A study comparing PCR to two direct bacterial cultivation tests in cases of known Lyme infection, found that the "results for 758 typical erythema migrans specimens showed positivity rates of 36% for MKP, 25% for PCR, and 24% for BSKII… CONCLUSIONS: Although possessing the potential to provide a rapid diagnosis, PCR is not more sensitive than culture for the direct detection of borrelia. Spirochaetes appear to be unevenly distributed throughout biopsy specimens, suggesting that diagnosis of Lyme borreliosis by direct detection of the causative agent in skin lesions is vulnerable to sample bias." (Picken, et al. A two year prospective study to compare culture and polymerase chain reaction amplification for the detection and diagnosis of Lyme borreliosis, *Mol Pathol* 1997 Aug;50(4):186-93).

There are a few other tests that show more promise. The three that show the most potential are the LDA, RWB, and the Phillips/Mattman. The Lyme Dot Blot Assay or LDA is used to detect the Lyme antigen in urine. It is available through IgeneX in Palo Alto, California. The company also tests for babesia and ehrlichia (www.igenex.com). The Reverse Western Blot or RWB is also used to test for antigen presence in urine. The two together have shown better outcomes in the diagnosis of Lyme than the Elisa and Western Blot. However, the best of the newer tests seems to be the Phillips/Mattman. According to a number of sources, it is 100% accurate—at least it appears to be from the preliminary data. (See for example: Phillips, Mattman, et al. A proposal for the reliable culture of Borrelia burgdorferi from patients with chronic Lyme disease, even from those previously aggressively treated, *Infection* 1998 Nov-Dec;26(6):364-7.) A similar type of testing is available through Bowen Laboratories—called the Rapid Identification of Borrelia burgdorferi or RIBb test—with results available within 24-48 hours (www.Bowen.org, see resource section). Another test that is showing usefulness, especially for chronic Lyme infection, is the Stricker NK Panel CD-57 test. It examines specific immunological markers to measure the effectiveness of treatment in chronic Lyme (see resource section).

Although other tests are sometimes being used—immunofluorescence assay (IF), antigen capture, spinal tap—many of the same problems occur as with the Elisa and Western Blot. The truth is that tests can help and, in some instances, confirm the diagnosis, but they are generally not very reliable (with the possible exception of the Phillips/Mattman).

In addition to poor tests, the difficulty for many practitioners with diagnosing the disease is that it is spreading out of what has been considered endemic areas. Infections are becoming more common along the West Coast and the southern potions of the U.S. In difficult cases, the diagnosis is best confirmed by working with someone with deep experience in Lyme infection (a Lyme-literate doctor or health care practitioner). An array of symptoms from the following list, living or visiting in an area where Lyme infection is common, and a Western Blot assay with at minimum two bands, one being 41kd and one other being Lyme specific, is an excellent indicator of infection. The IgG immunoblot seems to be slightly more accurate.

Symptoms of Lyme Borreliosis:

- Erythema migrans (EM) or bull's-eye rash (1/3 of those infected)
- Multiple EM lesions (in about 1/5 of those infected)
- Acrodermatitis chronica atrophicans (generally in late stage)
- Borrelial lymphocytoma
- Continual low-grade fever
- High fever, chills, or sweating (generally indicates bacterial coinfections)
- General flu-like symptoms
- Frequent headaches, neck stiffness
- Regular mild-to-moderate muscle and joint pain
- Severe unremitting headache (generally indicates coinfections)
- Bell's palsy (partial facial paralysis)
- Mental confusion or difficulty in thinking
- Disorientation, getting lost, going to wrong places
- Lightheadedness, wooziness
- Mood swings, irritability, depression
- Disturbed sleep
- Fatigue, tiredness, poor stamina

- Vision blurry or with floaters and/or light sensitivity
- Feeling of pressure in eyes
- Stiffness in joints or back
- Twitching of face or other muscles
- Neck creaks, cracks, stiffness, pain
- Tingling, numbness, burning or stabbing sensations, shooting pains
- Chest pain, heart palpitations
- Shortness of breath, cough
- Buzzing or ringing in ears, sound sensitivity
- Motion sickness, vertigo, poor balance
- Sudden hearing loss
- Tremors
- Weight gain or loss
- Swollen glands (can also be from coinfection)
- Menstrual irregularity
- Irritable bladder or bladder dysfunction
- Upset stomach and/or abdominal pain
- Glactorhhea

The Lyme Vaccine

A Lyme borreliosis vaccine, developed by SmithKline Beecham, arrived in late 1998. The first lawsuit due to damages caused by the vaccine was filed in December 1999. The vaccine was removed from the market in February 2002. The company cited lack of demand.

The primary problem with the vaccine is apparently that, in some people, it actually caused borreliosis and/or borreliosis symptoms. These included fatigue, arthritis, and cognitive problems. Case reports showed that from one tenth to nearly one third of the people vaccinated developed problems. A number of people who had had a previous Lyme infection experienced a reactivation of the disease in spite of previous antibiotic use for the condition. A study at Cornell University found that neurological symptoms such as neuropathy or cognitive impairment occurred in some people within two days to two months following vaccination. Of six patients studied two developed cognitive impairment, one chronic inflammatory demyelinating polyneuropathy (CIDP), one multifocal motor neuropathy, one had both cognitive impairment and CIDP, and one had cognitive impairment and sensory axonal neuropathy. Those with cognitive impairment had T2 hyperintense white matter lesions that showed during MRI scans. Other studies have found similar neurological impacts as well as arthritic activation.

CHAPTER TWO

Considerations in the Treatment of Lyme Borreliosis

To successfully treat Lyme infections, four simultaneous approaches are necessary: killing the spirochetes, immune modulation and support, collagenous tissue support, and symptomatic help. This kind of multi-pronged approach to disease treatment is not unusual, but it becomes more complex and needs to be more sophisticated with Lyme borreliosis because of the complexity and sophistication of the disease organism.

The treatment of Lyme infection by technological medicine is primarily limited to killing spirochetes. This is a common limitation of western medicine. In general, western approaches are rather blunt. They are concerned with kill (antibacterials), remove (surgery), reduce pain (opiates or the equivalent), reduce inflammation (corticosteroids), or force it do to what you want (hypotensives and so on). Subtle understandings of the complexity of physiological interactions and knowledge of how to enhance the responses of the body to disease are undeveloped. Recognition of and experience with the much more subtle palette of plant medicines in effecting these kinds of alterations and supportive interactions is either totally lacking or limited. Technologically-oriented physicians tend to be rather muscular and straightforward in their approach and to have little patience with "girlie men" approaches to healing. And with some conditions their approach is excellent, especially with trauma or acute conditions that need immediate resolution. For most everything else, outcomes from these western approaches and their heavy reliance on technological medicine are very limited. They are just not sophisticated enough to deal with the complexity of human beings as unique ecological expressions interacting with even more complex ecological environments. It is in these more complex areas that herbal approaches to Lyme infection really shine— that is, immune modulation and support, collagenous tissue support, and symptomatic help.

This is not to say that herbs are not useful as antimicrobials. Nonpharmaceutical approaches can also act to kill microorganisms and can be surprisingly effective. This is becoming especially true with the rise of antibiotic-resistant organisms such as the malarial parasite and multi-drug-resistant staph, both of which are eminently treatable with herbs and not by antibiotics.

Killing the Spirochetes

At this point in time, antibiotics are the clearest choice for killing spirochetes, with some caveats. Many people think of herbal approaches to treating Lyme borreliosis as "experimental." The term is meaningless in relation to Lyme disease. With Lyme infection *everything* is experimental. Antibiotics do work for many people but they do not work for all or even a large majority of those infected. The complexity of the organism's response and its ability to hide in the body in protected niches and to alter its form to resist antibiotic regimens make antibiotics useful but not a cure-all by any means. Because of the organism's complexity of response to host immune dynamics, antibiotics themselves remain experimental and the subtleties of their use are continually being developed as the disease itself is better understood. At this point in time, antibiotics are the most understood antispirochetals, the ones with which the most developmental work has occurred.

The major difference with antibiotics and other substances is that nearly the only substances tested for activity against borrelia organisms have been antibiotics. This presents problems in the development of herbal approaches to Lyme infection. There has been to date no testing of plant medicines for activity against Lyme borrelia.

Four factors were explored in deciding on the herbs used as anti-spirochetals in this book. (1) Did the herb show anti-spirochetal activity against other spirochetes; (2) Was there a long history of human use for spirochetal infections; (3) Did the herb show effectiveness for the particular symptoms of Lyme infection and/or for counteracting any of the complex physiological alterations that occur in the human body from Lyme infection; and (4) Have practitioners found it effective in contemporary use for Lyme infection and/or its particular symptom picture.

The herbs that fell into these four categories are the ones that are brought forward in this book as antispirochetals.

Immune Modulation and Support

The impacts that Lyme spirochetes have on the body and its physiological functioning are highly complex and far reaching. The organism can alter its genome structure and, consequently, its phenotype in response to environmental shifts. That especially includes the human body's immune responses to the organisms. The organism can affect any part of the body that possesses collagen tissues, which is pretty much any part of the body. But Lyme spirochetes do have favorite restaurants—the skin, central nervous system, and the joints, most often the knees.

Herbal medicines are especially good at dealing with the subtleties of the human immune response to spirochetal infection. I go into some detail on this in the pages that follow; it is impossible to talk meaningfully about Lyme infection and its treatment without doing so; the disease is just too complex to avoid it.

As an example, it is common to use astragalus for immune enhancement during Lyme infection. Astragalus is a good herb for this kind of condition, a very good herb in fact. But it is not enough to say that astragalus is good for immune enhancement during Lyme infection, because what the immune system does during Lyme infection changes depending on the length of the infection. In the beginning there is a reduction of Th1 response, due, in part, to the inhibition of the Th1 cascade by components in tick saliva. (Th1 levels can also be already low in the person prior to infection.) The higher or more healthy the Th1 response in the beginning of exposure to the spirochetes, the less chance there is of actual infection and the higher the likelihood that any infection that does occur will be mild. Astragalus is very good at enhancing the Th1 immune response and is essential if you live in an endemic area or have just been infected. However, late-stage Lyme, unlike many chronic infections, is not a Th2 dominant condition. It is Th1 dominant. And this contributes significantly to the auto-immune-like aspects of late-stage infections. The use of astragalus in late-stage Lyme has the potential of stimulating even further the Th1 response and thus worsening symptoms. Astragalus should not be used in late-stage Lyme infection.

As another example, overactive immune responses that cause severe inflammation in certain areas of the body, the eye for instance, can be adjusted by the use of location specific herbs to reduce that exact type of inflammation. In the case of Lyme-initiated uveitis, *Stephania tetrandra* is specific because of modes of activity unique to that particular plant.

So, the response to infection needs to be complex and based on a deep understanding of the disease progression, its particular actions in the body, and the subtleties of the herbs being used. Detail in discussing all this, for any sophisticated response to the infection, is inescapable.

Collagenous Tissue Support

The spirochetes cannot metabolize many substances on their own. They must scavenge them from their host. To do this, they have learned to use the host-immune system in very sophisticated ways. They use host-immune responses to not only to facilitate their spread through the body, to not only hide from host-immune responses themselves (by sequestering themselves within macrophages, for instance), but to help them get the food they need. They do this by using the host immune response to break down collagenous tissues in order to make a kind of soup of simpler substances from which they can extract their nutrients. Normally, in hosts with which they have a balanced, homeodynamic relationship, they remove collagens no faster than the host can replace them. Everybody is happy. But we are a newer species in this kind of a relationship. Even though they have infected us for millennia, these things take time to balance, and the spirochetes, at this point, tend to remove more collagen than most of us can stand and still remain healthy. So we have a lot of symptoms and these symptoms change, depending on where the spirochetes are scavenging collagen compounds. If it is in the brain, we have neurological symptoms. If the knee, arthritis sets in. To minimize these impacts, one of the best things to do is to lessen collagen breakdown and then enhance collagen replacement and healing throughout in the body. A number of herbs and supplements are highly specific for accomplishing these goals.

Symptomatic Help

While many of the specific symptoms that accompany Lyme infection will clear up with a competent course of antibiotics, three aspects of Lyme symptoms and antibiotic treatment are important to keep in mind. The first is that a competent antibiotic regimen may take up to thirty days for many people and that during that time, symptoms will persist or even worsen if Herxheimer reactions occur. The second is that for some people multiple antibiotic regimens or even lengthy, extended, antibiotic treatments are necessary. Lyme symptoms are a problem for these people and are often the reason they keep coming for more antibiotics. And third, for some people antibiotics do not work. Either the symptoms fail to resolve or they only partially resolve.

Herbal and supplement regimens can be designed for each of these groups to help protect the sites where symptoms are occurring, to reduce the symptoms, and to alleviate the suffering that accompanies Lyme infection. This kind of intervention can be remarkably effective. For example, devil's claw herb is exceptionally useful for the pain of Lyme arthritis and stephania root for reducing edema. And herbs are very effective in helping reduce the symptoms of post-Lyme-disease syndrome.

Especially important is the use of natural protocols for support during antibiotic therapies. The use of probiotics to help maintain bowel health or to correct bowel irregularities, such as candida overgrowth after extended antibiotic regimens, is essential.

Over time, as knowledge of Lyme infection and its myriad impacts deepens, these kinds of nonpharmaceutical interventions can become more highly sophisticated and effective. We are only at the beginning of our knowledge of this disease.

Update on the Protocol and Outcomes

As of June 2008 I have heard from about 500 people who have used this protocol, some 95% of them report complete or significant alleviation of symptoms. The online support group at www.planetthrive.com has several hundred questions and answers about the protocol and people's experiences with it. I highly recommend a visit.

Perhaps the main problem that practitioners have with the protocol is not clearly understanding the necessity for its alteration to fit the specific symptoms and ecology of each individual client. It is exceptionally important to realize that the Expanded Protocol, in Chapter Four, is an essential element of the protocol and that healing can often not occur without it. The use of eleutherococcus is crucial for those with severe fatigue; stephania is essential if eye or ear problems are present; a collagen support protocol is fundamental - healing is significantly retarded or impossible without it.

Perhaps the single most important herb is Japanese knotweed, secondarily cat's claw, third eleutherococcus. Andrographis is problematical. It is a good herb but may produce side effects. About one percent of people who take andrographis experience severe skin rash or hives that may take up to a month to resolve. About one percent of people experience taste problems from knotweed: metallic or bitter taste or even loss of taste. These problems will resolve upon discontinuing the herbs responsible.

The dosage guidelines are just that: guidelines. Some people need the highest dose for many months for the disease to clear, others have experienced significant help from just one tablet 3x daily of each of the herbs. Please adjust the dosages accordingly.

You can contact me at www.gaianstudies.org. Please write with any comments.

CHAPTER THREE

The Core Protocol: Natural Healing of Lyme Borreliosis

༃

*As they fell from heaven, the plants said
"Whichsoever living soul we pervade, that
man will suffer no harm."*

—THE RIG-VEDA

This core protocol is the heart of any comprehensive treatment of Lyme disease. It is the basic herbal regimen around which a full and comprehensive treatment plan can be developed.

This core protocol can be used along with antibiotic therapy and will increase the positive outcomes from antibiotics considerably. In terms of complementary treatment strategies, an antibiotic/core protocol approach will produce the optimum outcome for people who suffer infection with *Borrelia burgdorferi sensu lato* organisms and who wish to use antibiotics in their treatment. For practitioners, the numbers of people who do not respond to antibacterial protocols will decrease substantially with the use of this protocol and the incidence of post-Lyme-disease syndrome and/or chronic Lyme will decrease as well.

If antibiotics have not worked for you or your patients of if you do not desire to use antibiotics, then this core protocol will serve as the functional core around which a full treatment regimen can be designed. The three main herbs [and two supplemental herbs] in the core protocol—andrographis, Japanese knotweed (*Polygonum cuspidatum*) and cat's claw (*Uncaria tomentosa*) [astragalus, and smilax]—will significantly lower or eliminate spirochete loads in the body (including the central nervous system and brain), raise immune function in ways that will specifically empower the body to respond to borrelia infection (such as raising CD57 white blood counts), and significantly alleviate the primary symptoms of Lyme disease—brain fog and confusion, lethargy, arthritic inflammation, heart problems, and skin involvement.

The expanded protocol, which is outlined in chapter four, develops a more comprehensive herbal protocol that uses the core protocol as its central feature. It will significantly enhance outcomes if you (or your patients) are not using antibiotics or if antibiotics have previously failed to help. This expanded protocol can be used to adjust a nonantibiotic regimen to the particular symptom picture that exists with any particular Lyme patient.

The primary side effects of the core protocol are gastrointesintal upsets—generally nausea, upset stomach, and bowel sluggishness tending toward constipation. While all the herbs are extremely safe for use, three of the five herbs outlined in this section have GI-tract upset as potential side effects. These effects may be additive depending

---

THE CORE PROTOCOL

1. *Andrographis paniculata*, standardized to 10% andrographolides. 400 mg, 1-4 capsules or tablets 3-4x daily for 8-12 months.

2. Japanese Knotweed (Resveratrol): 1-4 tablets 3-4x daily for 8-12 months. The standardized tablets (e.g. those manufactured by Source Naturals, which I recommend) contain 1/2 gram (500 mg) of standardized Polygonum cuspidatum whole herb (Hu Zhang) and 10 mg of resveratrol.

3. Cat's claw (*Uncaria tomentosa*): 500 mg, 3-4 capsules 3-4x daily for 8-12 months.

Herbs that can be added to the core protocol

1. Astragalus, Dosage and use varies depending on stage of infection, see this chapter, after cat's claw.

2. Smilax (sarsaparilla): 425-500 mg, 1-4 capsules 3-4x daily for 8-12 months. See this chapter, after astragalus.

Please carefully read all dosage outlines, contraindications, and herb/drug interactions under each herb before applying this protocol.

on your (or your client's) particular constitutional make up. The dosage should be monitored carefully to minimize this and increased as the body adjusts to the herbs. *It is best to start at the lowest dose level and increase it weekly until the maximum dose is achieved. If gastrointestinal upsets occur, reduce the dose.* If the body adjusts well, the dosage levels can be increased more quickly. Vitamin C can be added to the diet (see next chapter) to both support collagen tissues and to counteract any tendency toward constipation.

A high dose range is necessary for the protocol to work well and, in my opinion, the best outcomes will occur with the use of encapsulated or tablet-form whole herbs rather than tinctures. I do have a bias toward whole herbs for most conditions. In any event, andrographis should not be used as a tincture—it is much too bitter. If you do use tinctures, the dosage range should equal that for the whole or standardized herbs outlined below.

The main contraindication for these herbs is pregnancy. There are a number of potential herb/drug interactions (astragalus is specific for certain stages of Lyme infection and not others, and so on), so the individual herb listings should be read carefully.

THE HERBS

ANDROGRAPHIS (*Andrographis paniculata*)

Common names: English: green chiretta (as opposed to sweet chiretta, which is another plant entirely), or andrographis (its primary English name in Western botanic practice). Also: chuan xin lian (TCM, China), senshinren (Japan), ch'onsimyon (Korea), kalmegh (ayurveda, Bengali), Maha-tita (northeastern India), Bhui-neem (India—because of its similar appearance, taste, and uses to Neem), Karyat (Hindi), Quasabhuva (Arabic), Kariyatu (Gujarathi), Nelaberu (Kannada), Nelacepu or Kiriyattu (Malayalam), oli-kiryata (Marathi), Bhuinimba (Oriya), Naine-havandi (Persian), Kalmegha or Bhunimba (Sanskrit), Nilavembu (Tamil and Telugu), and probably a whole lot more.

Family: *Acanthaceae.* Comprises 240 genera that includes 2200 species spread throughout Asia, Indo-malaya, Africa, South and Central America.

Part used: The above-ground, or aerial, parts of the plant are considered medicinal, though the root is sometimes (rarely) used in traditional practice.

Collection and habitat: Andrographis is part of the genus *Andrographis,* of which there are 28 species. They are primarily small annual shrubs many ranging (like andrographis itself) from one to four feet in height. Only a few of the species are medicinal, *Andrographis paniculata* being the most potent and commonly used.

This species is collected just before the plant blooms in early fall; the constituents in the plant are strongest at that time. Andrographis grows extensively throughout India, Pakistan, and Indochina, and is heavily cultivated in China, Thailand, East Indies, West Indies, and Mauritania. Its natural habitat is in evergreen and deciduous forests and along roadsides. It is especially common in hedgerows throughout the plains of India.

Cultivation: From seeds. Prefers full sun and warm climates (no snow and mild winters). Easily grown from seeds, it cultivates comfortably in all, including poor, soils. Grows well in indoor pots in any climate. The germination rate is 70%-80%.

Actions: Analgesic, anti-inflammatory, antibacterial, antiviral, antispirochetal, antifilarial, antimalarial, vermicidal, antitumor, antidiarrheal, antidiabetic, immune stimulant, hepatoprotective, cardioprotective, antithrombotic and thrombolytic, sedative, expectorant, hypoglycemic, depurative, choleretic.

Functions in Lyme disease: Andrographis is perhaps the best primary herb to use in the treatment of Lyme disease. It is antispirochetal, enhances immune function, protects heart muscle, is anti-inflammatory (helping with arthritic symptoms), crosses the blood/brain barrier where it is active as both an antispirochetal and calming agent, enhances liver function and protects the liver, helping clear infection from the body.

Because andrographis has shown significant protective effects against inflammation-mediated neurodegeneration in the brain it is essential to use in Lyme disease. It easily crosses the blood/brain barrier and accumulates in significant quantities in central nervous system tissues—brain, spinal cord, and cerebral spinal fluid.

Specific indications: Borrelia spp infection, with heart involvement, with arthritic inflammation, with low immune function, brain fog, confusion. Neuroborreliosis. Generally: any *Borrelia burgdorferi sensu lato* infection.

Plant chemistry: Andrographis makes a number of unique chemicals, among which are andrographolide, dehydroandrographolide, neoandrographolide, deoxyandrographolide, andrographoside, hydroxytrimenthoxyflavone, andrographine, homoandrographolide, andrographosterol, andrographane, andrographone, paniculide A, B, and C, and apigenin. Andrographolide is considered by most researchers to be the primary active constituent in the plant. It is highest in the leaves (about 2.5%), lowest in the seeds. Comprehensive studies, however, have shown significant synergistic activity between the plant's chemistries and in some clinical applications, andrographolide has been shown to be less active than the whole plant. Emerging concensus has decided that the four major andrographolides, that is, andrographolide, dehydroandrographolide, neoandrographolide, and deoxyandrographolide are all crucial constituents in the plant's medicinal actions. These are generally standardized to 10% in commercial extracts.

Radioactively labeled andrographolides have been used in clinical studies to track their movement in the human body. After 48 hours, andrographolides accumulate throughout the viscera. The concentration in various tissues has been found to be as follows: brain and spinal cord 20.9%, spleen 14.9%, heart 11.1%, lung 10.9% rectum 8.6%, kidney 7.9%, liver 5.6%, uterus 5.1%, ovary 5.1%, intestine 3.2%.

Excretion of the herb is initially rapid but then slows: 50% is excreted via the kidneys within two hours, 80% within eight hours, 90% within 48 hours. Because of its rapid excretion, the herb needs to be taken on a regular daily schedule.

Medical uses of andrographis: Andrographis has been used for

centuries in China and even longer in India where it is an indigenous
species. It has only recently entered western practice because of the
striking outcomes that have occurred in clinical studies conducted in
the East.

Ayurveda: In India, where it has the longest tradition of use (it appears
in texts 2000 years old), andrographis has been extensively used in
Ayurvedic, Siddha, and tribal practice. It has traditionally been used
for malaria, syphilis, as an antiwormer (anthelmintic), for dysentery
and bowel irregularity such as painful peristalsis and loose stools,
nerve pain (neuralgia), and sluggish liver. Its most powerful use has
been for either acute or chronic infectious diseases (as an antiperi-
odic), especially for influenza and chronic relapsing infectious diseases such as malaria, related borrelia infections such as East African
relapsing fever, worm infestations, leptospirosis, syphilis, and chronic
fatigue (i.e. general fatigue, debility, and weakness that will not
resolve). Andrographis was the primary remedy used in India during
the influenza pandemic of 1918, and is credited with reducing mortality rates from the disease.

Traditional Chinese medicine: In China, it is used for lung infections
and abscess, influenza-type illnesses, dysenteric disorders, painful urinary function, and leptospirosis. One of the specific indications for its
use is "fire toxin manifestations on the skin" such as sores, ulcerations,
or erythema migrans (EM)—the typical bulls-eye rash of Lyme disease. Considered a primary herb to clear heat, relieve fire toxicity, and
dry dampness especially for such things as damp-heat dysenteric disorders.

Western botanic practice: While andrographis was known to the nineteenth-century Eclectic practitioners, it was rarely used or imported.
Andrographis entered western practice in the latter half of the twentieth century and is becoming increasingly popular in Europe, especially in Sweden and the Scandinavian countries, for the treatment of
colds and flu. In the United States, the herb is now being used in combination with pharmaceuticals in the treatment of AIDS, and alone in
the treatment of colds and flu, and cancer. It is emerging as a potent
choice in the treatment of Lyme disease.

Scientific: The literature is extensive; this is a brief overview.

Andrographis shows powerful actions in the treatment of parasitic diseases. While Lyme disease is considered to be primarily a bacterial infection, the Borrelia spirochete (and all spirochetes) show strong similarities to parasites in their actions, appearance, behavior, and life cycle, and it is not surprising that andrographis has been found specific for them. The herb is active against leptospira spirochetes, has been used successfully in the treatment of leptospirosis, and more recently found by practitioners to be effective in the treatment of Lyme disease. Prior to the introduction of antibiotics, it was used successfully in the treatment of syphilis (another spirochete) in traditional Indian practice. Andrographis gels have been found effective for the treatment of periodontal disease organisms such as *Treponema denticola*, another type of spirochetal organism.

Clinical trials and studies have found andrographis to be active against a wide range of parasitical organisms: Plasmodium species (malaria), Leishmaniana species (leishmaniasis), *Wuchereria bancrofti* and *Brugia malayi* (filariasis), *Ascaris lumbriocoides* (human roundworm), *Dipetalonema reconditum* (canine parasitic worm), and leptospira spirochetes (leptospirosis). Many of these are, like Lyme, vector-borne diseases. Malaria and filariasis from mosquitos, leishmaniasis from sand flies, and dipetalonema from fleas. Leptospira organisms are excreted in the urine (generally by animals) and infection comes from contact with urine-infected water supplies. The organisms enter the human body through mucus membrane surfaces, by mouth, and through broken skin. Human roundworm infection is usually from food contaminated with roundworm eggs. Like borrelia organisms, the organisms involved in malaria, filaria, leishmaniasis, and dipetalonema use the chemical compounds injected into the new host by the vector through its saliva to facilitate entry and infection.

Andrographis's wide range of action can be seen by looking at the areas of the body infected by these parasitical organisms during the normal run of their diseases. Malarial parasites infect the blood and liver; dipetalonema infects dog connective tissues; leishmania organisms produce two forms of the disease, one in the skin, the other (more rare) in the internal organs. The internal organs affected are primarily the liver and spleen with organisms also circulating in the blood. Human round worms infect the intestinal tract. And of particular interest in the treatment of Lyme disease are the organisms that cause leptospirosis and filariasis, and the type of infections they cause in the human body.

In filaria infections, both *W. bancroftii* and *B. malayi* are similar organisms with identical vectors and exceptionally similar life cycles. *B. malayi* transmission occurs when the mosquito takes a blood meal from an infected host. The microfilaria enters the mosquito stomach and loses its sheath or outer coat some two hours later. The larvae then penetrate the gut wall and migrate to the thoracic muscles where, within 48 hours they moult into a stage 2 sausage-shaped worm. Two weeks later another moult occurs into the infective stage 3 state, a slender filariform larva. The larvae then migrate into the mosquito mouthparts where they wait for the mosquito to take a blood meal. They then pass out of the mosquito into the blood of the new host.

W. bancroftii exhibits a similar kind of periodicity as that of Lyme disease. The organisms only appear in the peripheral blood stream during the times that its mosquito vectors feed. At other times they sequester themselves in the internal organs, lodging themselves in the narrow capillaries in a static form. They shift their functioning depending on oxygen levels in blood and body temperature.

These two types of filaria can fill up the lymph system during their acute phases and eventually block it. The lymph is forced out of the system into the surrounding tissues, which causes fibrosis leading to the common name of the disease—elephantiasis.

Leptospirosis has many things in common with Lyme disease. Leptospira organisms infect over 160 mammalian species and different leptospira species have evolved to live within different mammal hosts. Wild animals act as a reservoir for the organisms through which domesticated animals are infected. Like borrelia spirochetes, leptospira organisms penetrate easily through denser, collagen-containing tissue.

After entering the body, the leptospires multiply in blood then spread to numerous other parts of the body, especially the kidneys and liver. Once in the kidney, the organisms migrate to the interstitium, renal tubules, and tubular lumen. They then move into skeletal muscle, endothelial tissue, the aqueous humor of the eye, the meninges of the brain and spinal cord, the cerebral spinal fluid, lungs, skin, and heart. In many respects, much like Lyme borreliosis organisms.

The symptoms, too, are much like Lyme: nonspecific flulike illness, fever, weakness, chills, myalgias, sore throat, cough or other pulmonary manifestations, mental confusion, meningitis, severe headache, cranial nerve palsies, encephalitis, mild delirium, brain fog, jaundice, diarrhea or constipation, nausea and vomiting, rash (macular, maculopapular, erythematous, urticarial, or hemorrhagic), floaters in the eyes, myocarditis, pericarditis, congestive heart failure, enlarged liver and spleen. Death is rare and usually from kidney failure.

Andrographis has been found effective for all these organisms, and is active in all the physiological systems that these organisms infect.

In clinical trials, 80% of leptospirosis patients treated with the whole plant or its isolated constituents were cured or experienced significant relief. The constituents used for treatment in non-whole-plant trials were deoxyandrographolide, andrographolide, and neoandrographolide in tablet form.

In vivo and *in vitro* studies have found andrographis extracts to be effective against malarial parasites. The extract used, composed of the four major andrographolides—deoxyandrographolide, andrographolide, dehydroandrographolide, and neoandrographolide—was found to be more effective than chloroquine in its effects. Deoxyandrographolide and neoandrographolide were found to be the most powerful constituents against malaria. Pretreatment with neoandrographolide for two weeks prior to infection enhanced treatment outcomes. The whole plant extract was found to be as effective as the separated constituents in another study; two weeks of pretreatment with the herb suppressed later infection with the parasite.

Dogs suffering from dipetalonema infestation were injected with a water infusion of andrographis. Worm clearance from the blood was 85% within forty minutes.

A trial with 32 people suffering from stage 3 filariasis found that 25 people who used the protocol experienced reductions in swelling and symptomology, seven experienced a worsening of symptoms. Andrographolide has been found to be specifically active against leishmanial parasites in *in vitro* and *in vivo* studies, "producing a normal blood picture and splenic tissue architecture."

A clinical trial with 80 people suffering acute bacterial dysentery found that andrographolide is exceptionally effective. Andrographolide (165 mg) was given three times daily over six days accompanied by rehydration therapy. Of the 80 patients, 66 were cured (82.5%), seven improved, and seven did not respond. Another trial of andrographolide, with 1,611 people suffering bacterial dysentery and 955 suffering diarrhea, showed 91.3% effectiveness. Andrographolide is especially effective with infectious *E. coli* bacteria.   Andrographis has also been found to be exceptionally active against *E. coli* enterotoxins—equivalent in its actions to standard pharmaceuticals; andrographolide being superior to loperamide for ST enterotoxin. As other researchers noted in similar studies, the herb "showed highly significant anti-secretory activity."

Chronic inflammation of the colon has responded well to enemas of the infused whole herb (combined with *Rhemannia glutinosa*) for a 14-day period; 61 of 85 patients were cured, 22 had symptomatic relief.

In vivo studies have found that andrographis has broad protective and healing actions for the heart and circulatory system. It inhibits arterial narrowing after angioplasty, decreases heart muscle damage after myocardial infarction, normalizes heart EEG readings, lowers blood pressure, inhibits noradrenaline induced hypertension, prevents clumping of platelets and thus clots in the blood vessels, and activates fibrinolysis—the process the body uses to dissolve clots.

Andrographis has been used in clinical trials testing its effectiveness in both hepatitis A and B infections. A marked improvement in symptoms and liver-function tests in the majority of patients was noted. In China, 83% of 112 people with hepatitis were successfully treated with whole-herb infusions. Other studies showed that andrographis whole herb combined with *Phyllanthus emblica* fruits (amalaki) taken three times daily for 30 days was effective in the treatment of viral hepatitis. The herb is directly effective against the hepatitis B virus *in vitro*. *In vivo* studies have shown a broad liver protective action by andrographis against a number of liver-damaging substances: carbon tetrachloride, alcohol, galactosamine, and paracetamol. Researchers noted: "treatment of rats with 400 mg/kg, ip, 1, 4, and 7 h[ours] after paracetamol challenge leads to complete normalization of toxin-induced increase in the levels of all the five biochemical parameters." Other *in vivo* studies found that andrographis and its extracts are potent stimulators of gall bladder function, bile flow, bile acids, and bile salts.

In a clinical trial with 129 people with acute tonsillitis, 65% of those treated with andrographolide showed significant improvements. In 49 pneumonia patients, 35 improved significantly and nine completely recovered. Another trial with 111 pneumonia patients and 20 bronchitis patients showed an effectiveness of 91% with the use of the whole herb. The addition of andrographolide to rifampin in the treatment of tuberculosis reduced mortality rates 2.6 times.

Andrographis has been found in studies to be as effective as nitrofurantoin in the treatment of pyelonephritis—infection of the kidney. Andrographis has far fewer side effects.

In vivo studies have shown that andrographis is strongly active against cobra venom, protecting mice from respiratory failure, increasing survival times considerably.

Andrographis has been found effective in clinical studies for infant cutaneous gangrene (study with 45 infants), leprosy (study with 112 people), herpes, chicken pox, mumps, neurodermatitis, burns, and vaginitis. An andrographis gel has been developed for gum disease in Europe; trials have shown it as effective as metronidazole gel in the treatment of periodontal disease. The andrographis gel has shown activity against a number of periodontal bacteria including

Porphyromonas gingivalis and *Treponema denticola* (another spiro-chetal organism).

The herb, in numerous studies, has shown general immune-enhancing activity—in essence, stimulating overall immunity and lessening autoimmune responses. Antibody production and phagocytosis is increased.

The herb has repeatedly shown mast-cell stabilizing and anti-PCA activity. PCA—passive cutaneous anaphylaxis—refers to allergic reactions in cellular tissue. Researchers note that the herb stops "inappropriate recruitment of macrophages to sites of tissue injury." The herb, as researchers commented, "significantly decreased degranulation of mast cells." Andrographolide has potent modulating effects on macrophage and neutrophil activity. The herb also extends this activity to the brain and central nervous system where it acts on microglia—basically brain macrophages. Andrographis has shown significant protective effects on inflammation-mediated neurodegeneration in the brain.

A number of double-blind trials have been conducted with the herb in the treatment of colds and flu. Consistent decrease in symptoms and improvement in recovery and recovery rates have been seen. The herb is often used in combination with eleutherococcus for this. Called Kan-Yang, it is a mixture of *Eleutherococcus senticosus* and andrographis. Researchers in a randomized trial with 53 children in Sweden note that "in early acute noncomplicated respiratory disease Kay-Yang tablets relieves considerably the treatment course and promoted cure." Two other studies—randomized, double-blind, placebo controlled—with 46 and 179 people respectively, found similar outcomes. Headache, malaise, nasal, and throat symptoms responded significantly to the herb. Taken to prevent the common cold, it showed significant activity in a randomized, placebo-controlled, double-blind study of 107 people. Dosage was 200 mg five days per week for the three winter months. The andrographis group had half as many colds.

The herb has been found to be active against the HIV virus *in vitro*, and useful in human trials in reducing viral load and increasing the lowered CD4 cell counts that exist in AIDS patients. Use of andrographis enhances AZT activity. Outcomes are better than with either alone.

It has also shown significant activity as an anticancer herb. In *in vitro, in vivo,* and in human clinical use, it has shown a broad activity against different types of cancers: anal, stomach, melanoma, skin, breast, prostate, colon, and leukemia. In a 1977 trial of 60 skin-cancer patients—41 with metastases—12 patients given andrographis alone recovered. All other patients were given andrographis along with standard drugs. There was no tumor regrowth in 47.

Basically, in Lyme disease, the herb does the following: (1) is antispirochetal; (2) protective and healing for neurological aspects of Lyme disease; (3) is specifically antiinflammatory for the central nervous system; (4) helps with other symptoms of Lyme such as pain, headache, confusion, and chronic fatigue; (5) stimulates the immune system to respond to the infection; (6) is cardioprotective; (7) modulates autoimmunity; (8) and because it is so broadly systemic it acts throughout the body to both protect the body from damage from spirochetes and kill them where they lodge, while at the same time offering a broadly systemic immune enhancement.

Dosage in Lyme disease: *Please read carefully.* Initial dosing: 1-4, 400 mg capsules 3-4x daily of a preparation standardized to 10% andrographolides. I suggest you begin with the lower dose for one week to allow your GI tract to get used to the herb. Gradually increase dosage to maximum, with increases of one tablet or capsule to the protocol every seven days, i.e. after seven days take two capsules 3x daily, then three, then four, then four capsules 4x daily. Maintain this dosage for at least 60 days. If GI-tract symptoms occur (nausea and so on) reduce the dose and allow your body more time to adjust. The amount of herb being taken can be reduced once Lyme symptoms decrease in severity, to three 400 mg capsules 4x daily and then to two 400 mg capsules 4x daily and so on. The herb should be taken for 8-12 months in the treatment of Lyme or until the disease is either under control or eradicated.

Note: Because of the severity of Lyme disease, its pervasive influence on multiple sites in the body, the organism's tenacity, and its deleterious effects on the central nervous system, I suggest the use of the standardized herb in the treatment of Lyme disease. These preparations normally contain 300 mg of standardized constituents and 100 mg whole herb—400 mg total. They come either encapsulized or in tablet form. I suggest capsules. The herb is exceptionally bitter and taking the tablets is unpleasant. The intensity of the impact as soon as they hit the tongue is astonishing.

The highest quality herb that is NOT standardized is available in bulk (one pound lots) from Raintree Nutrition. If you wish a non-standardized herb, I suggest this source; you may encapsulate it yourself if desired.

Note: Liquid tinctures of andrographis, when combined with other herbs in formula combinations in the treatment of Lyme disease, supply insufficient quantities of the herb and its very powerful andrographolides. While such formulations do help, their efficacy is much reduced.

Other preparation and dosage information: As a tonic, 400 mg 3x daily. In acute conditions, 1,000-2,000 mg 3-4x daily.

Older formulations were standardized to contain 4%-6% andrographolide. Newer ones are standardized for 10% of the four main andrographolides.

In traditional Chinese medicine, 9-15 grams of the non-standardized herb is used, usually in capsules, though sometimes granules of dehydrated tea are used. In India one half to one fluid ounce of the infusion is used for those who can stand the taste. The concentrated juice of the fresh plant is also used in India (10-60 minims) as is the tincture (one half to one fluid drachm). Traditional uses in India emphasize the expressed juice of the plant and water infusions. The whole plant is often blended with other herbs (e.g. cardamom) for use in GI-tract disturbances and, I suspect, for rendering it more amenable to consumption.

For diarrhea: decoction of 12 leaves of the plant in 8 ounces of water daily.

For dysentery or cholera: increase decoction intake to 3-5x daily.

Side effects and contraindications: Abortifacient: Not to be used during pregnancy. Contraceptive: Inhibits progesterone production. Not to be used by women when trying to conceive.

May cause mild constipation. Should not be used in active gall bladder disease. Very large doses may cause minor gastric upset. Very rarely: dizziness, heart palpitations, allergic reactions. **NOTE: About one percent of people using andrographis experience severe skin rash or hives which can take four weeks to clear once the herb is discontinued.** In a phase one, dose-escalating clinical trial with HIV positive and HIV uninfected volunteers, using pure andrographolide extracted from andrographis a number of side effects occurred. The dosage was high. It began at 5 mg/kg bodyweight for three weeks, then moved to 10 mg/kg bodyweight for three weeks, then to 20 mg/kg bodyweight for three weeks. The trial was suspended after six weeks due to side effects, including anaphylaxis. The dose of andrographolide, one of the four andrographolides in the plant, that was used ran from 500 mg to 700 mg per patient. With the dosing range suggested for Lyme, the amount of andrographolides is, at highest, 480 mg daily, with about 120 mg of that being andrographolide. In any case, **if dizziness, heart palpitations, or allergic responses occur, reduce dosage or discontinue the herb.**

One *in vivo* study with rats found that the herb lowered sperm production. Sperm production resumed normal levels upon discontinuance of the herb. Further studies did not confirm this result but because it exists in the literature, the herb is sometimes listed as antiandrogenic or antispermatogenic.

Herb/drug interactions: Andrographis may have a synergistic effect with isoniazid, a pharmaceutical used for tuberculosis.

CAT'S CLAW (*Uncaria tomentosa, U. guianensis*)
Common Names: Cat's claw, Una de Gato, Samento, Saventaro.
Family: *Rubiaceae*
Preferred species: *Uncaria tomentosa* but many of the others may work as well. Research data is incomplete.
Part used: Inner bark of the vine.

Collection and habitat: Cat's claw likes the jungle, the Amazon rainforest. It is a woody vine, sometimes of massive size and length that twists around trees, climbing up into the overstory in search of sunlight. It takes its name from the protruding, hook-like thorns on the vines.

Of the two primary South American species, *U. guianensis* grows throughout Peru, Bolivia, Brazil, Guyana, Paraguay, Trinidad, and Venezuela. *U. tomentosa* has a much wider range—Colombia, Ecuador, Trinidad, Guyana, Venezuela, Panama, Suriname, Guatemala, and Costa Rica.

The Ashaninka peoples of Peru are the largest commercial harvesters of the plant and supply many of the most reputable companies.

Note: Severe overharvesting is occurring in the Amazon in order to meet the industrialized nations' demand for the herb. Companies that utilize the root bark of the plant kill the plant. While the vine will die if it is completely debarked, it will resprout from the roots. One vine supplies a lot of medicine. In order to protect the plant populations, please buy only from companies that use the bark and not the root. The inner bark of the vine itself is highly active; the root does not need to be used. Outer bark preparations are not medicinally active.

Actions: Immune potentiator, immune stimulant, anti-inflammatory, antimutagenic, antitumor, antidepressant, antileukemic, antioxidant, antitumorous, antiviral, analgesic, anticoagulant, antidysenteric, blood cleanser and detoxifier, systemic tonic, diuretic, hypocholesterolemic, wound healer.

Actions in Lyme disease: Immune potentiator. Immune stimulant. Anti-inflammatory, analgesic. For central nervous system enhancement, cognitive impairments. Specific for arthritis and muscle pain in Lyme disease. As a general tonic for enhancing overall system health and sense of well-being.

Specifically, it increases CD57 white blood cell counts.

One of the best aspects of cat's claw for treating Lyme infection is that it raises CD57+ natural killer (NK) cells, a potent part of the immune system. Lyme spirochetes, after they become established in the body, specifically inhibit the production of this subset of the immune system. Low CD57 counts are a reliable diagnostic marker in chronic Lyme disease, especially that which will not resolve with the use of antibiotics. For those with chronic Lyme that presents with regular relapse accompanied by weakness and fatigue, cat's claw is especially indicated. This capacity of cat's claw to raise just this NK subset is one of the reasons why it has shown such good results in the treatment of chronic or late-stage Lyme infections. Using the herb to *keep* CD57 levels high helps inhibit the disease progression to late-stage or chronic status.

Specific Indications: Late stage Lyme infection, chronic Lyme, Lyme infection that does not respond to antibiotics. Especially Lyme disease with low CD57 blood count. Lyme arthritis. Lyme with chronic fatigue. Neuroborreliosis.

Plant chemistry: To date, cat's claw has been found to possess 17 different alkaloids, quinovic acid glycosides, flavinoids, sterol fractions, and numerous other compounds. More are being found all the time. A summary so far includes: oxindole alkaloids (both pentacyclic and tetracyclic), quinovic acid glycosides, beta-sitosterol, catechins, tannins, procyanidins, stigmasterol, campesterol, carboxy alkyl esters, ajmalicine, akuammigine, chlorogenic acid, cinchonain, coryantheine, corynoxeine, daucosterol, epicatechin, harman, hirsuteine, hirsutine, iso-pteropodine, loganic acid, lyaloside, mitraphylline, isomitraphylline, oleanolic acid, plamitoleic acid, pteropodine, rhynchophylline, iso-rhynchophylline, and their N-oxides, rutin, corynoxeine, iso-corynoxeine, rotundifoline, and iso-rotundifoline, speciophylline, strictosidines, uncarines A-F, vaccenic acid.

Medical uses of cat's claw: Although related uncarias have been used in both India and China for millennia, the South American species, especially *Uncaria tomentosa*, appear to possess more specific and potent actions for the immune system, on inflammatory conditions, and in the treatment of cancer. It is these South American species that all the shouting is about. However, many of the other species, especially the Chinese, are being tested and are being found to possess many of the same constituents and actions as *U. tomentosa*. They may prove to be as effective.

Cat's claw has been known to indigenous peoples in the Amazon for millennia. The Aguaruna, Ashaninka, Casibo, Conibo, and Shipibo tribes of Peru have used it extensively for treating asthma, inflammations of the urinary tract, arthritis, rheumatism, bone pain, child birth recovery, as a kidney cleanser, curing deep wounds, inflammation, gastric ulcers, treating tumors, diabetes, fevers, cirrhosis, internal cleansing, dysentery, general disease prevention, prostatitis, shingles, skin disorders, cancer, and, in a highly concentrated form, as a contraceptive.

Ayurveda: A related species, *Uncaria gambier*, is used in traditional Ayurvedic practice as a bitter astringent.

Traditional Chinese medicine: Two related species, *Uncaria rhynchophylla* and *U. sinensis* are used in traditional Chinese medicine. Other, similar species are used throughout China by traditional healers. Primarily they are used for damage to the central nervous system (e.g. epilepsy, seizures, tremors, convulsions); for dizziness and vertigo; to lower blood pressure; for eclampsia; for fever and headache; for liver disease. Many of these actions are also present in the Amazonian species such as *U. tomentosa*. The TOA alkaloids in all these species are specific for the central nervous system and have beneficial impacts on such things as epilepsy and tremors.

Western botanic practice: The herb is of recent introduction to the western medical world. The plant was unknown to the Eclectics, the great American botanical practitioners of the late nineteenth-century. The first non-indigenous accounts of the plant and its medicinal actions seem to have begun in the 1930s with a young Bavarian immigrant to Peru, Arturo Brell. Brell treated hundreds of people for cancer with the herb and in the early 1960s Brell shared much of his knowledge with an American professor, Eugene Whitworth. It was after Brell's death in 1974 that knowledge of the plant began to seriously engage western botanic practice, primarily from the work of the Austrian, Klaus Keplinger. In the late 1980s, knowledge of the plant began to catch on. Since the 1990s, it has found increasing use in the treatment of cancer, AIDS, immune disorders, and arthritis.

Scientific: The main reason that cat's claw has come to be of interest in the treatment of Lyme infections is that one study with Lyme patients found that the herb significantly alleviated symptoms of the disease and 85% of patients who were retested were found negative for Lyme infection. (Cowden, et al. Pilot study of pentacyclic alkaloid-chemotype of Uncaria tomentosa for the treatment of Lyme disease, December 28-2002-March 22, 2003. Presented at the International Symposium for Natural Treatment of Intracellular Micro Organisms (March 29, 2003) Munich, Germany.) This study is widely cited in literature and on the internet. However, in spite of the fact that cat's claw actually is good for treating Lyme infections, this study is seriously flawed and should not be cited so definitively.

To elaborate, 28 patients with advanced chronic Lyme borreliosis (all of whom had previously used antibiotics) were enrolled in the study. All patients tested positive using Western Blot. Half were placed in a control group that used conventional antibiotic therapy during the course of the study. Three improved, three worsened, eight showed no change in their condition. The other 14 patients received alternative treatments, one dropped out prior to study completion. Of the 13 patients who used cat's claw, 85% tested negative for borrelia after six months on the full alternative protocol and three quarters (or more) of all the patients reported improvements in nine parameters: fatigue, stomach pain, joint pain, memory problems, muscle pain, visual disturbances, emotional irritability, peripheral neuropathy, insomnia. This sounds great but on examination, a number of things are problematical with the study.

The people in the alternative treatment group used a variety of healing agents, not just cat's claw: a blood-type diet, enzymes with meals, enzymes between meals, vitamin and mineral supplements, laser detoxification, light-beam generator, skin brushing, bath detoxification, laughter, prayer, emotional release, **and** a TOA-free cat's claw supplement. The diets, enzymes, vitamin and mineral supplements are not defined as to type or dosage. Laser and bath detoxification, and so on, are, as well, not defined. Cat's claw dosage is not revealed. The study lasted six months, a preliminary report was given at the international conference in Germany after three months. In spite of diligent literature searches and e-mails to the study's initiator, I have been unable to obtain a full report of the study or an answer to a number of my questions (e.g., dosage).

What is interesting about the study is that it was with advanced chronic Lyme patients who had previously used antibiotics and all still tested positive for the disease. This population of people has been found to have low CD57 white-blood-cell counts and cat's claw specifically raises this particular subset. The inference is that the herb is effective. However, since so many other interventions were used along with the cat's claw, it is a useless study for the purposes of definitively stating (as I have seen some do) that in a clinical trial of 28 patients, cat's claw eradicated the disease in 85%. The study needs to be repeated with better controls and with cat's claw alone. Most of the other scientific literature is better, though none look at it specifically in the treatment of Lyme. What follows is merely a sample (Medline alone shows 135 listings for uncaria). An extensive list is available in the reference section.

In human studies, half the male volunteers (total numbers not stated) given a pneumonococcal vaccine also took a 350 mg capsule of C-MEd-100 twice daily for two months. C-Med-100 is a water-soluble extract of whole plant *Uncaria tomentosa* standardized to at least 8% carboxy alkyl esters. At five months, the volunteers were retested. A statistically significant immune enhancement was found in those taking cat's claw—elevation in lymphocyte/neutrophil ratios in peripheral blood and a reduced decay in the 12 serotype antibody titre responses to pneumonococcal vaccination.

Twelve human volunteers were separated into three groups, age and gender matched. For eight weeks, one group took a 250 mg tablet daily of C-Med-100, the second took a 350 mg tablet daily, and the third group took nothing. DNA repair after induction of DNA damage by a dose of hydrogen peroxide was tested. There was a statistically significant decrease of DNA damage and a concomitant increase in DNA repair in the supplement groups. There was also an increase in PHA-induced lymphocyte proliferation in the treated groups.

Thirteen people who were HIV positive and who refused to take conventional pharmaceuticals dosed with 20 mg of cat's claw daily for five months. White-blood-cell counts significantly increased. And another study, using cat's claw with AZT in the treatment of AIDS found that outcomes were better than with either substance alone, significantly reducing symptoms.

Of 45 people with osteoarthritis of the knee, 30 were treated with freeze-dried *Uncaria guianensis*, the remaining 15 with placebo over four weeks. Pain, medical and subject assessment scores, and adverse effects were collected at weeks one, two, and four. The antioxidant- and ROS-scavenging action of the plant were checked as well as its inhibition of TNF alpha and prostaglandin E2 production. No subjective or physiological side effects were found. Pain associated with activity and medical and patient assessment scores were all significantly reduced. TNF alpha and PGE2 were both inhibited, TNF alpha the strongest.

A randomized, double-blind, placebo controlled, 52 week, two-phase trial of a POA chemotype uncaria extract with 40 people, was conducted to assess its impacts in the treatment of rheumatoid arthritis. During the first phase, patients were treated with the extract or a placebo; the final 28 weeks all participants received the plant extract. There was a significant reduction of pain compared to placebo—the number of swollen and painful joints decreased.

Uncaria tomentosa extracts were used in the treatment of 273 people with different types of immune disturbances, including secondary immune deficiency after low-dose radiation exposure (84), immune deficiency due to chronic bacterial or viral infection (92), allergic reactions (55), and acute lymphoid leukemia and lymphatic leukemia (10). In those with low-dose radiation exposure, low CD4/CD8 ratios and suppressed NK cell activity improved, and so were CD3-CD16+ cell counts. TCR/CD3, HLA-DR, CD4 expression were all elevated after uncaria use. Monocytes exhibited integrins ICAM-1 and LFA3 expression and CD4+ cells exhibited LFA1.

The treatment of patients with immune deficiency due to chronic bacterial and viral infections found that the plant stimulated a normalization of immune response. There was a re-distribution of the cells in the CD8+ subset, an increase of antigen-dependent cytotoxic effector cells, and an increase in CD56 and CD57 expression on natural killer cells. Humoral immunity showed a decrease of previously elevated B-cell (CD+19 sIgM+) counts. The quantity of differentiated cells expressing surface immunoglobulin G and IgG serum concentration increased. There was a decrease in IL-2 receptor, transferrin, and HLA-DR expression. Phagocytosis was enhanced.

In vivo studies have found a wide range of action for uncaria species. Trials with the herb (and some of its alkaloids) have found that it exerts a beneficial effect on memory impairments induced by dysfunction of the cholinergic systems in the brain. These beneficial effects are partially due to the actions of the TOA alkaloids rhynchophylline and iso-rhynchophylline. The two POA alkaloids uncarine C and mitraphylline also helped but were much weaker in their effects than the TOA alkaloids.

Uncaria rhynchophylla was found to provide anticonvulsant effects in rats with kainic acid-induced epileptic seizures. The herb decreased lipid peroxide levels in the cerebral cortex.

The indole alkaloids hirsuteine and geissoschizine methyl ether were found to be significantly active in preventing chemically-induced epilepsy in rats.

Water extracts of *Uncaria tomentosa* (C-Med-100) were used to treat rats with chemotherapy-induced leukopenia. Neupogen-treated and untreated rats served as comparatives and controls respectively. Herb-treated rats received uncaria for 16 days; Neupogen (a pharmaceutical granulocyte colony stimulator) was given for 10 days. Both the C-MEd-100 and Neupogen groups recovered significantly sooner than the untreated group. The study (Sheng, et al. 2000) states:

> The recovery by C-Med-100 treatment was a more natural process than Neupogen because all fractions of white blood cells were proportionally increased while Neupogen mainly elevated neutrophils… other data showing enhanced effects on DNA repair and immune cell proliferative response support a general immune enhancement [by the herb].

Calves treated with whole herb *Uncaria tomentosa* (4200 mg per day for eight days) were examined (in relation to controls who received placebo) for changes in cellular immunity. The percentage of phagocytes in peripheral blood, their phagocytic index, and the values of random migration of neutrophils were significantly higher in treated calves than controls. There was a significant increase in the total number and percentage of CD2- T lymphocytes and CD4+ T helper lymphocytes and a decrease in WC4+ B lymphocytes, PMNL, and MID cells.

Another study examined the effects of *U. tomentosa* on experimentally induced pneumonia in calves. Calves were separated into two groups. One received placebo, the other 3600 mg per day for 17 days of a whole herb extract. In the treated group there was a significant increase in the total number and percentage of CD2+ and CD4+ cells. Temperature in the treated calves was lower. Researchers noted a "distinct inhibiting" of the synthesis and release of pro-inflammatory arachidonate (eicosanoids) and found it an effective modulator of the inflammatory process in the lungs of calves.

Both a freeze-dried water extract and a hydroalcoholic extract of *U. tomentosa* were tested for antiinflammatory actions against induced inflammation in rats. The hydroalcoholic extract was found more potent, NF-kappa B was inhibited.

U. tomentosa has been found to significantly reduce edema in arthritic rats. Its anti-inflammatory effects are slightly better than the pharmaceutical drug, indomethacin. The whole herb is significantly better as an anti-inflamatory than its isolated constituents. As usual, the whole plant's constituents posses synergistic actions.

It was found in studies with spontaneously hypertensive rats treated with uncaria extracts, that uncaria had a "protective effect for the endothelium against the influence of hypertension." Endothelium-dependent vasoconstriction decreased significantly in the treated group vs controls.

In vitro studies are numerous. The TOA alkaloids (from *U. sinensis*) rhynchophylline, iso-rhynchophylline, corynoxeine, and iso-corynoxeine and the indole alkaloids geissoschizine methyl ether, hirsuteine, and hirsutine were used to test for protective effects on glutamate-induced neuronal cell death in rat brain cells. Rhynchophylline, iso-rhynchophylline, iso-corynoxeine, hirsuteine, and hirsutine were found to be strongly protective of brain cells, preventing neuronal cell death.

Hirsutine and dihydrocorynantheine (from *U. rhynchophylla*) were found to have "direct effects on the action potential of cardiac muscle through inhibition of multiple ion channels, which may explain their negative chronotropic and antiarrhythmic activity." The chemicals' (concentration-dependently) decreased the maximum rate of rise and the prolonged action potential duration in atrial and ventricular preparations. In sino-atrial node preparations, cycle length was increased, slope of pacemaker depolarization was decreased, and there was a decreased maximum rate of rise and prolonged action potential duration.

A significant number of studies have found that uncaria extracts inhibit human cancer cell proliferation and induce apoptosis. This has been borne out in decades of successful use of the herb in clinical practice for various forms of cancer.

The plant has been found to possess immunomodulatory activity. It modulates the immunochemical pathways induced by interferon gamma, is a remarkably potent inhibitor of TNf alpha production, is an effective antioxidant, stimulates interleukin-1 and -6 production in alveolar macrophages, and stimulates phagocytosis.

The plant's quinovic alkaloids have shown antiviral activity, and broad anti-inflammatory actions.

Cat's claw is useful for Lyme infections in a number of areas: (1) For late stage or chronic Lyme infections it raises CD57 white blood cell counts; (2) It is an HLA-DR modulator; (3) It modulates the immune system, raising it where appropriate and lowering overactive responses where necessary; (4) It is antiinflammatory and reduces edema in arthritic conditions; (5) It helps with memory deficits and relaxes the CNS; (6) It helps protect the heart and heart function; and (7) It acts as an overall tonic to the system and enhances feelings of well being.

The TOA/POA controversy: If you begin looking into cat's claw for the treatment of Lyme infections, you will soon come across the product "TOA-free Cat's Claw." There is some amount of hysteria about this product. It is asserted that cat's claw products containing TOAs are not effective. *This is incorrect.* A review of the literature shows that a single series of *in vitro* studies—that is, in the laboratory, in test tubes only—found that the TOAs in a uniquely prepared solution of isolated cat's claw constituents, in some circumstances, had negative impacts on POA activity. Specifically what occurred was this: A blend of pentacyclic oxidole alkaloids—POAs—(28% pteropodine, 57% isopteropodine, 4% speciophyline, 6% uncarine F, 2% mitraphylline, and 3% isomitraphylline) was extracted from the herb and placed along with human endothelial cells in RPMI-1640 medium. This medium contained fetal calf serum, glutamine, penicillin, and streptomycin. This solution was allowed to stand for seven days to produce supernatants, basically a liquid layer floating above the solid matter, which was filtered and then stored for use in testing. This liquid was then used to determine the activity of the POAs on a number of things such as endothelial cells and normal B and T lymphocytes. One of the tests run with this supernatant found that it caused "a yet to be identified factor" to be produced by endothelial cells which caused an increase in "normal resting or weakly activated human B and T lymphocytes." The study's next sentence, confusingly, states: "In contrast, the proliferation of B and T lymphocytes and Raji and Jurkat cell lines is significantly inhibited" (Wurm, et al, 1998).

A supernatant of tetracyclic oxindole alkaloids (TOAs) was also prepared along the same lines as the POAs, containing 67% rhynchophylline and 33% iso-rhynchophylline. It was found that this supernatant "acted antagonistically" on the release of the "as yet to be identified factor" and, in a dose-dependent manner, reduced the effect of the POA supernatant in Raji and Jurkat cells. Raji cells are human Burkitt's lymphoma B lymphocytes, Jurkat cells are leukaemic cells. These are abnormal cancer cells tested under unique laboratory conditions. No generalization can legitimately be made from this except, perhaps, that TOAs inhibit POA impacts on certain cancer cell lines *in vitro.* To reliably make that point, the study would have to be repeated by other researchers. It has not.

Two papers were published outlining this same series of tests. Both are by very nearly the same group of authors. The tests themselves were cited in three other publications. These five papers are the ones continually cited as a justification for the statement that TOAs inactivate POAs.

No other researchers have found these kinds of results; the tests themselves have never been duplicated by another laboratory and they alone do not justify the statement that TOAs inactivate POAs. Additionally, the papers are inconsistent in their statements (and very unclear in their reasoning and structure). As noted above, the POA supernatant caused an increase in "normal resting or weakly activated human B and T lymphocytes. In contrast, the proliferation of B and T lymphocytes and Raji and Jurkat cell lines is significantly inhibited." It both increases and inhibits, according to the authors, the proliferation of B and T lymphocytes.

The TOA supernatant acted to inhibit the release of the unknown lymphocyte proliferation factor and reduced the POA supernatant inhibition two cancer cell lines. That is all the studies (appear to) show in any event. This is a far cry from showing that TOAs inhibit the action of POAs in the human body. No legitimate generalization about the herb's impacts on immune function can be made by this study.

The TOAs used in the study are incomplete to the plant. Only two were used—rynchophylline and iso-rynchophylline. The plant also contains their N-oxides, corynoxeine, iso-corynoxeine, rotundifoline, and iso-rotundifoline. Additionally, the amounts of the two TOAs used exceeds that found in the plants themselves; these were isolated constituents taken out of their plant matrix and purified. Within the whole plant, synergistic actions occur between the many plant chemicals. There is no evidence that in whole plant form these TOAs inactivate anything.

Scores of other studies in five countries, including the research for five patents, have shown that the whole herb (which naturally includes TOA alkaloids) stimulates the immune response.

Other studies have found that the TOA alkaloid iso-rhyn-chophylline, which naturally occurs in the plant and which was one of those whose supernatant was tested, stimulates immune function, specifically phagocytosis.

None of the many other researchers working with the plant the past 25 years in scores of studies found that the naturally occurring TOA alkaloids inactivated the naturally occurring POAs. The majority of all studies on the plant have been conducted using the whole herb or other proprietary formulations that contain both TOAs and POAs.

As only one example, researchers using a water extract that does contain both TOA and POA alkaloids tested the growth inhibitory effects of the uncaria preparation C-MED-100 on a human EBV-transformed B lymphoma cell line—that is, Raji cells. This is the same cell line as discussed in the study above. These researchers found, however, that the "Raji cells were strongly suppressed in the presence of the C-Med-100." (Sheng, et al. Induction of apoptosis and inhibition of proliferation in human tumor cells treated with extracts of Uncaria tomentosa. *Anticancer Res* 1998 Sept-Oct; 18(5A):3363-8.) So, a similar study with the whole-plant extract found that the TOAs did not inhibit POA action on that very same cell line.

Some researchers make the point that there are at least two (some say three) types of *Uncaria tomentosa* plants that grow in the Amazon and that natives distinguish between these types. This is true. The natives routinely harvest the type that contains the most POAs for making medicine. However, the plant they harvest and have been using for millennia, naturally contains *both* POAs *and* TOAs. This naturally occurring POA/TOA-containing herb has been successfully used for a very long time by these indigenous peoples to enhance immune activity. Additionally, the herb has been successfully used in clinical practice with thousands of people for over half a century in South America to enhance immune response. No people using the herb have found that the TOAs inactivate the POAs; the whole herb, containing both TOA and POA alkaloids, is effective in actual practice. This is why scientists became interested in it.

Of additional concern for the TOA/POA study discussed is that two of the paper's authors hold the patent on the process for removing TOAs from POAs and may possibly have, as well, an interest in a company that makes TOA-free cat's claw.

Without extensive *in vivo* studies and other laboratory replication of this original study, it is improper to determine that TOAs inactivate POAs in cat's claw. The evidence from other studies and millennia of use indicates that the assertion is incorrect.

The herb itself, without any fiddling around, will work exceptionally well, especially for Lyme disease. In part, this is because the two different types of oxindole alkaloids offer a two-pronged impact on Lyme symptoms. The POAs enhance immune function, mainly the immunologic system cells, particularly those responsible for non-specific and cellular immunity. The TOAs mainly affect the central and peripheral nervous system, helping with the neurological impacts of Lyme infection. *TOAs and POAs are both important in Lyme infection.* There is no need to seek out a TOA-free extract. You will, as well, save a great deal of money. The TOA-free extracts are, compared to the natural herb, exceptionally expensive.

The quinovic acid controversey: A rumor has spread that the quinovic acids in cat's claw are, at root, the same as quinolone antibiotics. The rumors say that this is why cat's claw is effective against Lyme spirochetes. Concern has been generated by this untrue assertion because quinolone antibiotics, in some instances, can cause severe inflammation in tendons. So, the word is that cat's claw can cause tendonitis, resulting in tissue destruction over time. This is all completely untrue. The quonovic acids in cat's claw are structurally different than quinolone antibiotics. Molecularly, they are not the same at all and they do not do the same things.

Dosage in Lyme disease: *Please read this carefully.* One to four 500 mg capsules 3-4x daily for 8-12 months. Begin at lowest dose and increase incrementally every seven days, i.e., after seven days take two capsules

3x daily, then three capsules 3x daily, then four 3x daily, then four 4x daily. Maintain this dosage range for 60 days minimum. If desired, dosage can then be slowly decreased as Lyme symptoms subside. If symptoms worsen as dosage is lowered, increase dosage. This dosage modification minimizes chances of GI-tract upset upon initially taking the herb (see Side effects).

- If necessary, dosage can be increased beyond this suggested range. Dosage for active arthritic conditions ranges from 3-5 grams daily. Therapeutic doses for other acute conditions ranges from 2-3 grams 2-3x daily up to 20 grams a day.

- I strongly suggest the use of Raintree cat's claw only (www.raintree.com). It is the primary supplement on the market that I know is of high quality and ethically wildcrafted.

- *Do not take this herb while taking stomach acid blockers as they may inhibit the conversion of the herb into its active form in the stomach.*

- If taking a liquid extract, the lighter the color of the tincture, the more potent it will be.

- Some practitioners suggest that the tincture should not be taken sublingually as some evidence exists that it needs to be activated by stomach acid. Add the tincture to six ounces of water and one teaspoon of lemon juice or apple cider vinegar to increase the bioavailability of the herb.

Side effects: Dosages of 3-4 grams of the herb at a time have sometimes caused intestinal upset such as loose stools, diarrhea, and/or abdominal pain. These effects tend to subside as the herb is used over time. Lower the dose of the herb if you experience these side effects. Discontinue use if diarrhea persists longer than three days.

Contraindications: Do not use if you have had an organ transplant or are using immunosuppressive drugs. Do not use if you are trying to become pregnant. Do not use if you are using blood thinning medications or are scheduled for surgery. Cease use of the herb 10 days prior to any surgery.

Herb/drug interactions: Do not take with stomach acid blockers or antacids such as PeptoBismol, there is some concern that they can inactivate the herb. Do not use with immunosuppressive drugs such as cyclosporin. The herb may potentiate the action of coumadin and other blood thinning drugs.

JAPANESE KNOTWEED (*Polygonum cuspidatum*)

Common names: (English) Bushy or Japanese knotweed and (sometimes) Mexican bamboo or Chinese knotweed, Hu Zhang (Chinese), kojo and itadori (Japanese), hojang (Korean).

Family: *Polygonacae*

Part used: The root (rhizomes).

Collection and habitat: Native to Japan, North China, Taiwan, and Korea, the plant is an invasive botanical that, it has been discovered, is exceptionally hard to eradicate. Introduced as an ornamental in 1825 in Britain and the U.S. in the late 1800s, it is now naturalized throughout much of mainland Europe, the British Isles, Canada, New Zealand, and at least 36 states in the United States. Apparently, all the plants in Europe are females and clones, making the plant, as the Japanese Knotweed Alliance comments, "one of the biggest females in the world in biomass terms." A new concept of measurement.

The plant does look a little like bamboo, though the leaves are considerably different. It grows to a height of 3-9 feet (1-3 meters). The roots (rhizomes) are collected in the spring or fall and dried for use.

Cultivation: Easily, and primarily, from pieces (minuscule) of the rhizomes/roots—the easiest form of propagation. Seed cultivation is difficult as male plants with fertile pollen are rare outside Japan and China. It forms dense thickets and is an especially good planting for erosion control in industrial-damaged ecosystems and in volcanic areas (so they say). It is a potential plant in phytoremediation work as it tolerates and removes copper from copper-contaminated soil and concentrates it in its roots. The plant likes to live along the edges of streams so pieces of the root can be carried off during floods, where they then spread with gleeful abandon. Considered an invasive species, it is diligently attacked with evangelical fervor by Native purists who will often stop by your home, uninvited, to share their insights on eradication. The plant cultivates internal strength in any who grow it intentionally and is a powerful addition to the western botanical pharmacopoeia.

Actions: Antibacterial, antiviral, antischistosomal, antispirochetal, antifungal, immunostimulant, immunomodulant, antiinflammatory, angiogenesis modulator, central nervous system relaxant, central nervous system (brain and spinal cord) protectant and anti-inflammatory, antioxidant, antiathersclerotic, antihyperlipidemic, antimutagenic, anticarcinogenic, antineoplastic, vasodilator, inhibits platelet aggregation, inhibits eicosanoid synthesis, antithrombotic, tyrosine kinase inhibitor, oncogene inhibitor, antipyretic, cardioprotective, analgesic, antiulcer (slightly reduces stomach acid and protects against stress ulcers), hemostatic, and astringent. The plant can be eaten and is a good source of vitamin C, making it a good antiscorbutic. Both shoots and leaves are eaten.

Functions in Lyme disease: A broadly systemic plant, Japanese knotweed modulates and enhances immune function, is active against a number of gram-negative and gram-positive bacteria including leptospira and *Treponema denticola* spirochetes, is anti-inflammatory for both arthritic and bacterial inflammations, protects the body against endotoxin damage, helps reduce Herxheimer reactions, and is a cardioprotector.

As mentioned earlier, one of the main factors in the emergence of Lyme arthritis is the spirochetal-stimulated release of a number of particular compounds called matrix metalloproteinases (MMPs). The most common are MMP-1, -3, and -9. Production of MMP-1 and MMP-3 in Lyme arthritis occurs through a particular grouping of pathways—mitogen-activated protein kinases (MAPKs), specifically c-Jun N-terminal kinase (JNK), p38 mitogen-activated protein (p38), and extracellular signal-regulated kinase 1/2 (ERK 1/2). MMP-9 production occurs through the JNK pathway and another, the protein kinase C-delta pathway.

While there are a number of herbs that can reduce autoinflammatory conditions stimulated by MMP-1 and -3 (e.g. curcumin), the only herb that specifically blocks MMP-1 and -3 induction through these three particular pathways is *Polygonum cuspidatum.* Resveratrol (one of the plant's constituents) is also directly active in reducing MMP-9 levels through both the JNK and protein kinase C-delta pathways; it has been found to specifically inhibit MMP-9 gene transcription. Another component of the plant, rhein, inhibits the JNK pathway for MMP-1, -3, and -9 expression.

Polygonum cuspidatum's constituents cross the blood/brain barrier where they exert actions on the central nervous system: antimicrobial, anti-inflammatory, as protectants against oxidative and microbial damage, and as calming agents. The herb specifically protects the brain from inflammatory damage, microbial endotoxins, and bacterial infections.

Knotweed enhances blood flow especially to the eye, heart, skin, and joints. This makes it especially useful in Lyme as it facilitates blood flow to the areas that are difficult to reach to kill the spirochetes. It is a drug and herb synergist, facilitating the movement of other herbs and drugs into these hard-to-reach places when taken with them. It is specific for Lyme skin manifestations, especially in reducing or eliminating skin responses to Lyme disease—both the typical EM rash in the U.S. and that of acrodermatitis chronica atrophicans, which is common in European Lyme disease. It is also specific for treating bartonella coinfections that can occur in Lyme disease (see chapter five).

Specific indications in Lyme disease: Neuroborreliosis, bulls-eye rash, acarodermatitis chronica atrophicans, low immune function, spirochete infection, Lyme arthritis, endothelial damage from Lyme and Lyme coinfections, cardiac involvement, post-Lyme-disease syndrome, bartonella coinfection.

Plant chemistry: Emodin, chrysophanol, rheic acid, emodin monomethyl ether, polygonin, physcion glucoside, piceid, resveratrol, transresveratrol, polydatin, glucofragulin, physcion, fallacinol, citeroosein, questin, questinol, protocatechuic acid, catechin, dimethylhydroxychromone, napthoquinone, methylcourmarin, and numerous flavinoids, polysaccharides, and condensed tannins.

Medicinal uses of Japanese knotweed: Part of the importance of Japanese knotweed as a new medicinal useful in clinical practice, is understanding that invasive plant species are specifically indicated for use with invasive or emerging diseases such as Lyme, West Nile encephalitis, SARS, hepatitis C, HIV, and so on. The use of invasive species of plants in treatment reduces the impact on non-invasive medicinals and begins using plants that are accompanying invading pathogens as they move into new ecoregions.

While there is a long historical use of the plant in Asia, especially China and Japan, stretching back 2000 years, there has been little knowledge of the plant in the western world until recently. Research on and subsequent use of the plant as a phytomedicinal has been primarily because of its high content of resveratrol, a potent vasodilator and inhibitor of platelet aggregation (among other things). Interest in the compound was stimulated by the French "paradox." That is, they ate lots of cheese and still had really low cholesterol counts and little incidence of heart disease while we in the United States were dying like flies. This was found to be due, in part, to their high intake of red wine. (In the U.S., researchers make haste to say this does not mean you should drink. In France they smile and continue to sip their wine.) A number of compounds have been found to play a role in this "paradox" but resveratrol and trans-resveratrol seem to be the most potent. Red wine, particularly that made from pinot noir grapes, contain significant amounts of these compounds, especially trans-resveratrol. The compounds easily move across the gastrointestinal mucosa and circulate in the blood stream. They cross, as well, the blood/brain barrier. Some 131 patents have been granted in the U.S. on the herb and its constituents for treating a variety of conditions, primarily cancer, inflammations, and neurodegenerative diseases.

It should be stressed that while resveratrol does do amazing things, it, by itself, is not sufficient in treating Lyme disease. The whole herb is crucial. Other constituents of the plant, such as emodin, polydatin, and trans-resveratrol have all been found to be "wonder-drugs" in their own right. As usual, depth research is showing that the plant constituents possess broad spectrum actions and synergistic actions that the single chemicals do not. As a whole herb it is much more powerful than any constituent used alone. As only one example, while resveratrol is strongly active against *Neisseria gonorrhea*, even antibiotic resistant strains, it is only active against this one neisseria species. The whole plant is active against many others.

Ayurveda: This particular species has not been used in traditional Ayurvedic practice though 11 other species of polygonum are, many used similarly to the Japanese knotweed of TCM practice.

Traditional Chinese medicine: In traditional Chinese medicine the herb is used for invigorating and clearing the blood, and for its antipyretic, detoxicant, anti-inflammatory, antirheumatic, diuretic, expectorant, antitussive, and stasis eliminating and channel-deobstructant actions. Primarily, it is used in the treatment of jaundice, rheumatic pain, strangury with turbid urine and leukorrhea, dysmenorrhea, retained lochia, bleeding hemorrhoids and anal fissure, wounds and injuries, scalds and burns.

Other uses include respiratory infections and damage to skin: burns, carbuncles, skin infections, snakebite (usually as a poultice), bacterial dysentery, acute infectious hepatitis with jaundice, hepatitis B (surface antigen positive) chronic active hepatitis, neonatal jaundice, cholelithiasis, cholecystitis (with damp heat or severe heat syndrome), trichomonas, bacterial vaginitis, hyperlipidemia, and psoriasis. (Basically, it is used to treat pathogenic heat in the blood, cough from lung heat, constipation from accumulated heat in GI tract, jaundice and liver inflammation due to damp-heat, accumulated heat in skin.)

Western botanic practice: This particular herb was unknown to western botanic practice until recently (and is still unknown to most American and European botanic practitioners). The Eclectics knew of and used (to some extent) nine polygonum species, primarily *Polygonum hydropiper*—water pepper. Many of them possess actions similar to that of Japanese knotweed, though they cannot be used in a simple substitution for this particular polygonum species. Japanese knotweed is distinctly unique in a number of respects.

Scientific: Surprisingly, given how unknown this plant is to western botanic practice, there are literally hundreds of studies on the plant and its constituents. In the west these studies have primarily focused on the actions of resveratrol, followed (in descending order) by the whole plant, and the constituents: trans-resveratrol, emodin, and polydatin. The scores of clinical and laboratory studies in China have been primarily on the whole plant and the single constituent polydatin. For the best overviews of the studies on the plant and its constituents see Pervaiz, S. Resveratrol:from grapevines to mammalian biology, *The FASEB Journal.* 2003, 17:1975-1985; Ignatowicz, E. and Baer-Dubowska, W. Resveratrol:a natural chemopreventative agent against degenerative disease, *Polish Journal of Pharmacology*, 2001, 53:557-569; and Chang, H. and But, P. *Pharmacology and Applications of Chinese Materia Medica*, Volume 2, NJ:World Scientific, 1987, 733-740.

In vitro studies have found a broad antibacterial action by the plant and its constituents against such organisms as leptospira and *Treponema denticola* spirochetes, *Staphylococcus aureus, S. albus, Neisseria cattarrhalis, N. gonorrhoeae, N. meningitidis,* A and B Streptococci, *E. coli, Proteus vulgaris, Pseudomonas aeruginosa, Salmonella typhi,* and *Shigella flexneri.* Part of its action as an antibacterial comes from inhibiting bacterial DNA primase.

The herb is also broadly antifungal (part of resveratrol's function in the plant). It is strongly inhibitive against *Candida albicans.*

In vitro studies have found a broad antiviral activity against a number of viruses including respiratory syncytial virus (RSV). Asian influenza (type A), herpes simplex, and ECHO 11 (enteric cytopathic human orphan) viruses were inhibited by a 10% water decoction of the whole herb. ECHO viruses, previously thought to be benign (where the word "orphan" comes in), are now known to cause a number of diseases including: rashes, diarrhea, respiratory infections (cold, sore throat, bronchitis, bronchiolitis), muscle inflammation, meningitis, encephalitis, and pericarditis (inflammation of the membrane around the heart).

In other studies, a 2% water decoction of the plant strongly inhibited adenovirus type III, poliomyelitis virus type II, coxsackie A and B viruses, encephalitis B, HIV, and the ECHO11 group viruses. A 20% water decoction had a significant inhibitory action against hepatitis B antigen, decreasing HBAg titer by eight times.

In vivo and *in vitro* studies found the herb and the single constituent polydatin to have a potent antitussive action as well. (The antiviral effect against respiratory viruses and this antitussive effect make the herb exceptionally useful for use during upper respiratory infections, including SARS.)

The herb has been used for a long time in China for the treatment of burns. It has been found in clinical trials to promote scabbing (eschar formation) and inhibit bacterial infections in the damaged skin. The herb reduces exudation, prevents water and electrolyte loss, and hastens wound healing. In one study, 60 people with second- and third-degree burns were treated with the herb—10%-71% of the body surface was burned, 15 were suffering skin infections. The second-degree burns healed in four to six days, third-degree in 20-42 days. Other studies reveal similar outcomes. Reduced scarring and less tissue death is common with the use of the herb for burns. This comes in large measure from its powerful angiogenesis modulating (blood vessel generating and controlling) actions.

In burned skin, blood clots (thrombosis) within the capillaries lead to necrosis of the underlying tissues. Vasoconstriction, slow blood flow, and damage to underlying blood vessels are key conditions leading to thrombosis in burned skin. Clinical studies in China using special microscopes found that Japanese knotweed acted as a microcirculatory stimulant. It stimulated the blood flow into burned skin, expanded the blood vessels, stimulated the healing old blood vessels, and initiated the development of new ones.

Japanese knotweed is an angiogenesis *modulator*. That is, it stimulates the formation of new blood vessels and the healing of damaged ones in areas such as burned skin. But it also stops the development of new vessels and blood flow in areas where it should not occur, such as in malignant and benign tumor formation. It is a classic tonic herb in this respect and the only one I am aware of for maintaining the blood vessels themselves. It has, as part of this mode of action, specific modulating and protectant actions on the endothelial cells that line blood vessels.

Polygonum acts as an angiogenesis stimulant in a number of ailments: burns, chronic inflammations such as rheumatoid arthritis, debilitating opthamlic disorders such as diabetic retinopathy and macular degeneration, brain disorders such as stroke, and various forms of heart disease such as coronary artery disease and angina. It acts powerfully as an angiogenesis inhibitor in both benign and malignant tumors. It may also come to soon play an important role in the treatment of a certain form of macular degeneration (MD), so-called wet MD in which the growth of abnormal blood vessels occurs in the eye.

In studies of heart disease, researchers found that resveratrol, one of the primary components of polygonum, protected the cardiovascular system against ischemic-reperfusion injury, promoted vasorelaxation, protected and maintained intact endothelium, was antiatherosclerotic, inhibited LDL levels, was an antioxidant, and suppressed platelet aggregation. Chinese researchers found that the constituent polydatin was also broadly active in the cardiovascular system. They noted that it strongly stimulated vasorelaxation throughout the body, including the bronchial capillaries.

Polydatin is especially effective in treating burn shock, enhancing cardiac and microcirculatory functions. It restores decreased cardiac functions: output and stroke volume index. It restores pulse pressure to normal, decreases the number of adhesive white blood cells, and the amount of open capillaries returns to near normal. The degree of damage to scorched lung tissue was alleviated. It inhibits multiple-organ failure from burn shock.

In vitro studies have found that the water extract of the whole herb markedly decreases cellular cholesterol content. Specifically, polygonum inhibits cholesterol ester formation in human hepatocytes by inhibiting acylcoenzyme A-cholesterol acyltransferase. The main active constituent for this was found to be resveratrol. However,

Chinese researchers found that polydatin also possessed strong actions, significantly lowering cholesterol levels within seven days.

In vivo studies of polydatin and the whole herb on the cardiovascular system found that the herb markedly increases contraction amplitude levels even while lowering blood pressure. Coronary flow is increased while coronary resistance is significantly decreased. Both polydatin and the whole herb enhance cardiac and microcirculatory functions and restore decreased cardiac functions. Resveratrol has also been found to possess similar actions. It inhibits tissue factor expression in vascular cells in response to pathophysiological stimuli, including bacterial, thus reducing inflammation in the heart and vascular tissue. It normalizes vascular endothelium.

The whole herb and its constituent, resveratrol, are both strong antioxidants. People who consume red wine or the herb have been found to have significantly increased antioxidant activity in their blood. This potent antioxidant action has been detected throughout the body. Interestingly, resveratrol seems to be an antioxidant modulator in that it will increase antioxidant action when needed (most of the time) but will lower it in instances where necessary, e.g. in leukemia cells.

Resveratrol is a potent inhibitor of the dioxygenase activity of lipoxygenase. Lipoxygenase is involved in the synthesis of mediators in inflammatory, atherosclerotic, and carcinogenic processes. By its potent inhibition of the dioxygenase activity of lipoxygenase, both the herb and resveratrol have pronounced effects on inflammatory processes such as arthritis, cholesterol levels in the blood, and cancer.

In part this is because resveratrol blocks eicosanoid production. Eicosanoids are powerful, very short-lived, substances—quasi-hormones if you will—that are generated from three different fatty acids: dihomogammalinolenic acid, arachidonic acid, and eicosapentaenoic acid (EPA, common in fish and fish oils). Arachidonic acid is the predominate generator in mammals, being stored in cell membranes. Through cyclooxygenase (COX) enzymes, arachidonic acid is transformed into potent pro-inflammatory and platelet-aggregating thromboxanes and inflammatory prostaglandins. Through lipoxygenase (LOX) enzymes it becomes the potent inflammatory, and white blood cell stimulating, leukotrienes, hepoxillins, and lipoxins. The herb inhibits both LOX and COX pathway inflammations.

Resveratrol specifically inhibits the generation of arachidonic acid metabolites. These metabolites are involved in a number of autoimmune and allergic reactions, in tumor development, and in psoriasislike conditions of the skin. Not surprisingly resveratrol causes a dose dependent inhibition of the biosynthesis of prostaglandin E immunoreactive material.

Recent research has found that the plant and its constituent, resveratrol, interfere with the actions of nuclear factor-kappaB (NF-kB). This transcription factor is strongly linked to inflammatory and immune responses. It is active in the regulation of cell-proliferation and apoptosis, cell transformation, and tumor development. It controls the gene expression of cytokines, chemokines, growth factors, and cell adhesion molecules, some acute phase proteins, including the inflammatory mediators iNOS and COX-2. Bacteria such as Lyme spirochetes can activate NF-kB, causing a cascade of immune-mediated cellular reactions. The herb apparently modulates the actions of NF-kB rather than acting simply as its suppressor. Resveratrol also modulates interferon-gamma-induced neopterin production and tryptophan degradation.

The herb, in fact, is a potent immunomodulator. It normalizes immune response, especially in diseases where autoimmune reactions are stimulated (such as Lyme disease and Lupus). It seems able to bring up immune function when necessary and reduce its local manifestations when overstimulated, e.g. in rheumatoid arthritis. This is a very strong aspect of the plant's actions.

As an example of its stimulatory actions, knotweed has been found to raise white blood cell counts during radiation and chemotherapy. It was effective in treating leukopenia or low white blood cell counts in 67 people undergoing radiation and chemotherapy for tumors. Of the 59 who had no break in radiation treatment,

40 had an increase in white blood cell count (WBC) of 100/mm3. Of the eight who had a break in radiation treatment seven showed the same increase in WBC.

The herb also stimulates the formation of fibroblasts. These undifferentiated cells migrate to injury sites, especially (in this case) in the skin and collagenous tissues, and undergo alterations to form new cells necessary for healing. In arthritis and psoriasis, the herb reduces inflammation and stimulates the production of new fibroblasts and their translocation to the areas of damage.

Good therapeutic outcomes were found in China in a clinical trial of the herb for 100 people with rheumatic arthritis, rheumatoid arthritis, lumbar hypertrophy, and osteoarthritis. The herb has been found to be especially effective in acute inflammatory diseases such as appendicitis, appendiceal abscess, tonsillitis, and pneumonia. In 45 people with pneumonia who were treated with the herb, body temperature dropped to normal in 1-1.5 days. In 26 cases of acute appendicitis, 14 cases of appendiceal abscess and four cases of perforated appendix complicated with peritonitis, all were cured by a decoction of the whole herb. Clinical studies have also found the herb to be effective in acute icteric viral hepatitis, inflammation of the bone and bone marrow, psoriasis, herpes, and cervix erosion.

In cancer studies, plant constituents from knotweed, primarily emodin and its derivatives—citreorosein, emodic acid, physcioin, fallacinol, chrysophanic acid, and rhein—were found to be potent oncogene signal transduction inhibitors through inhibiting protein-tyrosine kinase and protein kinase C. Another constituent, resveratrol, acts to inhibit tumor growth, metastasis of tumors, and angiogenesis in cancer. Resveratrol inhibits DNA synthesis in cancer cells (specifically Lewis lung carcinoma) and inhibits the binding of vascular endothelial growth factor to human umbilical vein endothelial cells. This constituent of the herb reduces the new blood vessels being created by cancerous clusters eventually cutting off their supply of blood. Resveratrol has been found to be a significant inhibitor of cancer formation *in vitro* and *in vivo* for both mouse mammary gland and skin cancers. Dose-dependently, resveratrol inhibited up to 98%

of skin tumors in mice; the percentage of mice with tumors, at the highest dose range, was lowered by 88%.

Resveratrol affects cancer at three stages of its life cycle: initiation, promotion, and progression. It inhibits metastases, cuts off tumor blood supply, and helps normalize cell differentiation. It is strongly antimutagenic.

The constituents, resveratrol and trans-resveratrol, are also considered to be phytoestrogens, useful in the treatment of menopausal symptoms. Resveratrol increased bone mineral content, mass, and density in postmenopausal women who received just 100 micrograms daily. It binds to estrogen receptors, thus enhancing estrogen activity in the body. A number of studies have found that neither of these two constituents of the plant seem to exacerbate estrogen-sensitive cancers. In fact, resveratrol actually inhibits human breast cell cancers. Resveratrol may act as more of an estrogen modulator in that it has been found to be both agonist and antagonist for estrogen receptors alpha and beta.

Harvard Medical School researchers recently found that resveratrol duplicates the life-extending benefits of caloric restriction. Reducing daily intake of calories by up to 40% dramatically extends life span and slows down aging in laboratory studies with different lab animals. Resveratrol has been found to mimic these effects in yeasts, flies, worms, mice, and in *in vitro* studies on human cells. It apparently turns on sirtuins, genes that are stimulated during times of low food availability (or fasting). These genes slow down human aging through a number of mechanisms and they are present in nearly all life forms that have been studied. Japanese knotweed contains a number of SIRC chemicals (sirtuin activating compounds) that initiate this process in living organisms. The most potent appear to be resveratrol and trans-resveratrol.

The herb and its constituent have also been found to enhance and potentiate the action of other drugs and herbs when taken with them.

Japanese knotweed and its constituents also possess strong actions in the central nervous system and brain, and this range of activity is where a great deal of interest in the plant is being generated.

Knotweed and the constituents, trans-resveratrol and resveratrol, have been found to be strongly neuroprotective through a variety of actions in numerous studies. One of the herb's mechanisms of action in this regard is as an antioxidant. Resveratrol and trans-resveratrol have been found to protect rat embryonic mesencephalic cells from a powerful pro-oxidant, tert-butyl hydroperoxide. Another study found that regular use of trans-resveratrol prevented streptozotocin-induced cognitive impairment and oxidative stress in rats (an Alzheimer's-like condition). And yet another found that trans-resveratrol protected and reversed many of the impacts of induced stroke in rats.

While the herb's antioxidant actions are important, trans-resveratrol, for example, has been found in a number of studies to strongly protect neuronal structures from damage through mechanisms other than antioxidant activity alone. Resveratrol has been found specific for protecting the brain from neurotoxic substances such as the B-amyloid peptides, which are associated with Alzheimer's disease.

Resveratrol and trans-resveratrol are specific for reducing inflammation in the brain and central nervous system. In spinal cord injuries resveratrol "remarkably" reduced secondary spinal cord edema, significantly suppressed the activity of lactate dehydrogenase, reduced malondialdehyde content in the injured spinal cord tissue, and markedly improved NA+, K+- ATPase activities. It immediately stimulates microcirculation to the injured tissues.

Low-level, chronic inflammation in the brain and central nervous system plays a major role in many neurodegenerative conditions. Both the herb and its constituents are specific for such inflammations. They have been found active for such things as: amyotrophic lateral sclerosis and other motor neuron diseases, Parkinson's disease, Alzheimer's disease, bulbar atrophy, dementia, Huntington's disease, myasthenia gravis, stroke, multiple sclerosis, fronto-temporal dementia, encephalomyelitis, traumatic brain injury, cerebral ischemia, and so on. The resveratrols specifically protect brain cells from assault, whether chemical or microbial in origin. The herb and its constituents, as well, stimulate microcirculation in the brain.

At least four patents have been granted on this herb's constituents for neurodegenerative disease treatment. *In vitro* and *in vivo* studies have found the resveratrols effective for a number of these conditions. Some clinical reports support these findings and a number of clinical trials are underway.

Thus, the herb has a number of specific actions in the treatment of Lyme disease: (1) stimulating microcirculation, esp. to the eye, knees, heart, and skin which helps carry active constituents to those locations to affect spirochete presence; (2) reducing inflammation in tissues, thus lessening both skin and arthritic impacts from the spirochetes; (3) protecting and correcting heart function and reducing inflammation in heart tissue, especially helping with symptoms associated with Lyme carditis: lightheadedness, shortness of breath, palpitations, and chest pain; (4) reducing autoimmune reactions to Lyme; (5) wide-spectrum antibiotic/antiviral action, including against spirochetes; (6) immune enhancement; (7) acting as a synergist with other herbs or drugs in the treatment of Lyme; (8) protecting endothelial integrity from Lyme spirochetes and Lyme coninfectious agents such as bartonella; (9) reducing reactive oxygen species production in the central nervous system and brain.

Dosages in Lyme disease: *Please read carefully.* Commercial forms of the herb are available as a partly standardized preparation or it can be used whole as a tea or decoction. The commercial forms, usually tablets, are the easier ones to use in Lyme infection.

Standardized tablets: One to four tablets 3-4x daily depending on severity of symptoms. Begin at the lowest dose and increase incrementally every seven days, that is, after seven days take two tablets 3x daily, then three tablets 3x daily, then four tablets, 3x daily, then four tablets 4x daily. Maintain this for at least 60 days. As symptoms decrease in severity the dosage can be incrementally lowered to a maintenance dose. Maintain use of the herb for 8-12 months or until symptoms or infection is resolved. If symptoms worsen upon lowering the dose, increase.

The standardized tablets (e.g. those manufactured by Source Naturals, which I recommend) contain one half gram (500 mg) of polygonum whole herb (Hu Zhang) standardized to 8% total resveratrols and 10 mg of resveratrol. This formulation is titled "Resveratrol" on the bottle. But not any old resveratrol will do. Make sure that whichever kind you buy includes the whole plant in some form, standardized or not, in at least this amount.

Whole herb: The whole herb can be prepared as a decoction or encapsulated to take in whole form. In whole form: powder well and take 8-16 double-ought capsules daily in four equal doses. As a decoction: one ounce herb (28 grams) in 32 ounces (1 litre) water, simmer for 20 minutes, strain, cool, and drink in four equal doses during the day. Incrementally increasing the dose with these whole-herb preparations is a good idea as well.

Other dosage information: TCM dosage is 9-30 grams of the whole herb daily taken internally in whole form or as a decoction. For burns, anal fissures, etc.: soak a cotton ball in a strong decoction of the herb and apply topically throughout the day or soak a burn dressing in the decoction and apply.

Contraindications and side effects: While a very safe herb, Japanese knotweed is contraindicated in pregnancy. Side effects of high dosages are primarily gastrointestinal in nature—dry mouth, bitter taste in mouth, nausea, vomiting, abdominal pain, diarrhea. The toxic dose is high, about 75 grams for a 150-pound (75 kg) person. Large doses are often used. Up to 1000 mg daily of resveratrol are being used in ongoing clinical trials for its effects on HIV infection.

Note: If gastrointestinal side effects occur, reduce the dose.

Herb/drug interactions: Should not be used with blood-thinning agents. Discontinue use of the herb 10 days prior to any surgery.

ASTRAGALUS (*Astragalus membranaceous* or *A. membranaceous* var. *mongholicus,* aka *A. mongholicus*)

Family: *Leguminosae*

Common Names: Astragalus (English), Huang-Qi (Chinese)

Part used: The plant is a perennial with a long, fibrous, root stock. The root, which is the part used for medicine, is often found thinly sliced and dried (a traditional preparation in Chinese medicine) and most closely resembles a yellow tongue depressor. Bulk quantities of the powdered or coarsely ground organic root are commonly available through herbal suppliers to western botanic practitioners.

Habitat: There are over 2,000 species of astragalus in the world, 16 of which grow in the United States. The leaf structure looks like a typical member of the pea family. It is a short-lived, sprawling perennial, and grows up to four feet in size.

Astragalus is native to northeast China, although it has been planted a great many other places, including the United States. Wild populations are still rare in the west, although it is under cultivation as a medicinal in the United States and escape to the wild is inevitable.

Cultivation and collection: Astragalus is started from seeds in the early spring indoors. The seed coat needs to be scored with something like sandpaper prior to planting. Growers (e.g. Elixir Farm) have found that it prefers a sunny location with "deep, sandy, well-drained, somewhat alkaline soil. It does not like mulch or deep cultivation. The crowns of the emerging plants are very sensitive to compost and respond well after they have gained some momentum in the spring." Not surprisingly, given the plant's medicinal actions, it is highly resistant to insect damage, crown rot, mildew, and drought.

The plant grows larger and more woody each year, the roots are harvested beginning the fall of the third year or spring of the fourth. Spring and fall harvests occur in China.

Actions: Immune enhancer, modulator, stimulant, and restorative; antiviral; antibacterial; adaptogen; tonic; antihepatotoxic; diuretic; enhances function in lungs, spleen, and GI tract; heart protector; hypotensive.

Function in Lyme borreliosis: Immune potentiator and modulator. Increases interferon-gamma and interleukin-2 levels. Enhances CD4+ counts and balances the CD4/CD8 ratio. Astragalus is specific for immune atrophy and enhances function in spleen and thymus.

Studies with tick-borne Lyme infection in mice found that if interferon-gamma and interleukin-2 levels were stimulated in the animals prior to tick bite, the rate of infection by borrelia spirochetes was much lower than otherwise. The reduction of these immune complexes, especially interleukin-2, is stimulated through components in the tick saliva. Keeping levels high will significantly reduce the likelihood of infection. If infection does occur the impacts of the disease will be significantly lessened, symptom development will be milder, the whole thing easier to cure. The herb should be taken year-round if you live in a Lyme-endemic area.

Other studies have found that, during Lyme infection, the higher the CD4 white blood cell levels the better the individual response to infection and treatment. High CD8 levels appears in a number of studies to promote the disease process. Lower CD4 counts correlated to increased spirochete load and spirochete clustering in joint and skin. Increased CD4+ levels are essential for immunological control of spirochetal load. Astragalus will raise CD4+ cells counts and balance the CD4/CD8 ratio. Basically, the herb increases the Th1 response.

The herb is also indicated for Lyme borreliosis with heart involvement. It both inhibits the development of and corrects the left ventricular dysfunctions that can occur in Lyme infections, enhances heart function, reduces palpitations, and alleviates angina. (It is specific for palpitations with shortness of breath.) It is an anti-stressor (adaptogen), helping reduce the impacts of stress (including stress from infection). It is an anti-fatigue agent, specific for chronic fatigue. It is effective for night sweats. It is helpful for many neuroborreliosis symptoms (tingling, paralysis, and numbness).

Specific indications in Lyme infection: Residence in an endemic area, low immune function, chronic fatigue, night sweats, Lyme carditis (angina, palpitations, shortness of breath), Pre-, early, and early-disseminated Lyme borreliosis infections, ehrlichia coinfection. Not suggested for use in late stage borreliosis. (See "Contraindications.")

Plant chemistry: Astragalosides 1-7, astraisoflavin, astramembranagenin, astrapterocarpan, bea-sitosterol, betaine, formonetin, GABA, isoastragaloside 1, 2, and 4, isoliquiritigenin, linoleic acid, linolenic acid, soyasaponin-I, kumatakenin, choline, glucaronic acid, 4'-hydroxy-3'-methoxyisoflavone 7, a couple of dihydroxydimethylisoflavones, 3'-hydroxyformonentin, calcium, folic acid, choline, copper, iron, magnesium, manganese, potassium, sodium, zinc.

About astragalus: Astragalus, first mentioned in the 2,000 year old Chinese text *Shen Nong Cao Jing*, is considered to be one of the superior tonic herbs in Chinese medicine. It has developed into one of the primary immune herbs used worldwide over the past four decades.

Ayurveda: Five species of astragalus are used in the materia medica of India, none of them this species. They are minor herbs used primarily as emollients.

Traditional Chinese Medicine: Astragalus has been a major herb in Chinese medicine for between two and four thousand years. Its traditional uses are for spleen deficiency with lack of appetite, fatigue, and diarrhea. It is specific for disease conditions accompanied by weakness and sweating, stabilizes and protects the vital energy (qi), and is used for wasting diseases, numbness of the limbs, and paralysis. Other uses: tonifies the lungs, for shortness of breath, frequent colds, and flu infections; as a diuretic and for reduction of edema; for tonifying the blood and for blood loss, especially postpartum; for diabetes; for promoting the discharge of pus; for chronic ulcerations, including of the stomach; and sores that have nor drained or healed well.

Western botanic practice: The herb was not used in western botanic practice until the tremendous east/west herbal blending that began during the 1960s. It is now one of the primary immune tonic herbs in the western pharmacopoeia.

Scientific: A considerable amount of scientific testing has occurred with astragalus. This includes clinical trials and both *in vivo* and *in vitro* studies. Medline lists 799 citations for studies with astragalus, and this does not include the many Chinese studies that have never been indexed for Medline. Two U.S. patents have been granted for the use of astragalus for immunostimulation. What follows is merely a sampling.

Immune function: Most of the clinical studies and trials regarding immunostimulation have been focused on the use of astragalus in the treatment of cancer and/or as an adjunct to chemotherapy to help stimulate chemo-depressed immune function. A number of other studies have examined its immune effects with a range of different conditions.

The herb has been used with children suffering tetralogy of Fallot after radical operations to correct the condition. Tetralogy of Fallot is a complex of four heart abnormalities that occur together, generally at birth. Surgery is used to correct it. Astragalus was found to decrease abnormal levels of IgG, IgM, C3, C4, CD8+, and CD19+ while increasing levels of CD4+ and CD56+. The ratios of CD4/CD8, CD3/HLA-DR, and CD3/CD16 normalized between the second and third week of use. IL-6 and TNF-alpha both began decreasing in the first week and by week four were in the normal range.

When used in the treatment of herpes simplex keratitis, levels of Th1, including IL-2 and IFN-gamma, increased and Th2 levels, including IL-4 ad IL-10, decreased showing that the herb modulated Th1 and Th2 levels. This same kind of effect has been found in the treatment of numerous cancers. For example, in a study of 37 lung-cancer patients, astragalus was found to reverse the Th2 status normally present in that condition. Th1 cytokines (IFN-gamma and IL-2) and its transcript factor (T-bet) were enhanced and Th2 cytokines were decreased.

In clinical trials with a number of different cancers and congestive heart conditions, astragalus has been found to increase CD4+ levels, reduce CD8+ levels, and significantly increase the CD4/CD8 ratio. The plant has been found to have a broad immunostimulatory effect. Use of the herb with cancer patients undergoing chemotherapy found that white blood cell counts improved significantly (normalizing). The herb has been found to be specifically useful in preventing or reversing immunosuppression from any source—age, bacterial, viral, or chemical. Phagocytosis is enhanced and superoxide dismutase production from macrophages is increased.

Heart disease: There have been numerous clinical trials with the herb for treating heart disease. It has been found specific for inhibiting coxsackie B infections, both as an antiviral and as a heart protector. It will reverse damage to the heart in a number of conditions. With respect to Lyme carditis, probably the most important are its impacts on left ventricular function, angina, and shortness of breath. While it is not completely protective for atrioventricular block, it does improve electrophysiological parameters and ameliorates AV block to some extent.

In a trial of astragalus for two weeks with 19 people with congestive heart failure, 15 people experienced alleviation of symptoms of chest distress, dyspnea, and their exercise tolerance increased substantially. Radionuclide ventriculography showed that left-ventricular modeling and ejection fraction improved, HR slowed from 88.21 to 54.66 beats/min.

Forty-three people suffering from myocardial infarction were tested with astragalus. Left-ventricular function strengthened. The ratio of pre-infection period/left ventricular injection time decreased. Superoxide dismutase activity in red blood cells increased and lipid peroxidation of plasma was reduced.

In a study with 316 cardiac patients with various cardiomyopathies (angina, myocardial infarction, arrhythmia, myocarditis), astragalus was found to be effective when compared to lidocaine and mexilentine (which were not found effective). With astragalus, the duration of ventricular late potentials shortened significantly.

In the treatment of 92 patients suffering ischemic heart disease, astragalus was more successful than nifedipine. Patients were "markedly relived" from angina pectoris. EKG improved 82.6%.

Anti-inflammatory activity: Astragalus has been found to possess anti-inflamamtory activity by inhibiting the NF-kB pathway and blocking the effect of interleukin-1 beta in leukotrine C production in human amnions. The constituent astragaloside IV inhibits increases in microvascular permeability induced by histamine. The whole-herb decoction has been found to reduce capillary hyperpermeability.

Neurological actions: Astragalus has been found to improve anisodine-induced memory impairment on memory acquisition and alcohol-elicited deficit of memory retrieval. After use of the herb, the number of errors were reduced. The plant has been found to exert potent antioxidant effects on the brain, helping to prevent senility.

Fatigue: Astragalus has been found effective in alleviating fatigue in heart patients and in athletes. Twelve athletes were randomly separated into two groups, and six were given astragalus. Astragalus was found to positively influence anaerobic threshold, enhance recovery from fatigue, and increase fatigue threshold.

Hepatitis: A number of trials have found the herb effective in the clinical treatment of hepatitis B and liver disease. Liver function is improved, protected from damage, and regeneration is stimulated.

Astragalus preparations: Many astragalus formulations are standardized, although I'm not sure that the literature really supports standardization with this herb. The root is usually standardized for either 0.4% or 0.5% 4'-hydroxy-3'-methoxyisoflavone 7, but the reasons are not exactly clear for doing so. No literature exists that I can find that lays out why in fact this particular constituent was singled out and not the astragalosides. (Astragaloside IV, for instance, is the one of the primary active ingredients of the plant for heart disease. It increases exercise tolerance and reduces chest distress and dyspnea, and optimizes left ventricular function.) The methoxyisoflavone constituent for which the plant is standardized is an anabolic-type compound that enhances strength and muscle formation and may have some protective actions in upper respiratory infections and on digestive function. Data on its functions are somewhat unclear and hard to come by. I have been unable to locate any clinical or laboratory studies on the constituent, although they must exist somewhere. Their rarity stimulates speculation.

In any event, for ease of use and quality of herb, I would suggest the Planetary Herbs formulation which contains 500 mg standardized root and 500 mg whole root in combination. The whole root contains constituents that are essential for carditis and enhanced immune function. And, indeed, the majority of the Chinese studies—clinical and laboratory—were with the whole herb.

Dosage in Lyme disease: Astragalus is an essential herb to use all year long at tonic doses if you live in an endemic area. It is exceptionally useful during active infections, especially during early and early-disseminated stages.

Tonic dose: For preventing Lyme infection or lessening disease impacts in case of infection: 1,000 mg 2x daily (Planetary Herbs formula or equivalent).

Active Lyme infection: Use along with the core protocol. Begin with 1,000 mg 3x daily and work up to 4,000 mg 4x daily for at least

60 days, then decrease if desired to a lower dose. Take for 8-12 months.

Note: You may buy the powdered whole herb in pound (.4kg) lots and encapsulate it yourself or take it in juice. Tonic dose: 3 "00" capsules 2-3x daily or up to three tablespoons of the powder in juice. For active infection take six "00" capsules 3-4x daily or up to six tablespoons daily of the powder in juice.

Contraindications: *Please read carefully.* During tick bite, the tick releases compounds in its saliva that stimulates Th2 while inhibiting Th1 immune responses. This has effect of reducing interferon-gamma and interleukin-2 levels in the body to which the spirochetes are specifically sensitive. The Lyme spirochetes take advantage of this to invade and colonize tissues. As the body adjusts, it begins stimulating Th1 responses and, eventually, Lyme infection becomes a Th1 dominant disease (rather than Th2 as are many chronic conditions). The spirochete has, however, had time to adjust and, in spite of enhanced Th1 response, it is well established and uses numerous techniques to avoid Th1-mediated destruction. (Th1 levels do help keep spirochete load lower than would otherwise occur. Reducing Th1 response, e.g. interferon-gamma, will severely increase disease symptoms. However increased Th1 levels not only decrease spirochete load but, in late stage infection, exacerbate Lyme symptoms such as arthritis.)

With late-stage Lyme infection, astragalus is contraindicated as it will stimulate already overstimulated Th1 responses. This may have the impact of worsening disease symptoms. *Astragalus is not indicated in late stage Lyme borreliosis.* However, it is highly indicated, and very specific, for use in pre-, early, and early disseminated Lyme infection.

Herb/drug interactions: Synergistic actions: Use of the herb with interferon and acyclovir may increase their effects. The herb has been used in clinical trials with interferon in the treatment of hepatitis B and outcomes were better than with interferon alone. It has also shown synergistic effects when used with interferon in the treatment of cervical erosion; antiviral activity is enhanced. Drug Inhibitor: Use of the herb with cyclophosphamide may decrease effectiveness of the drug. Not for use in people with organ transplants.

SMILAX (*Smilax glabra* and other Smilax species)

Common names: In English, sarsaparilla or smilax. Tu fu ling (Chinese), dobukurya (Japanese), t'obongnyong (Korean), dwipautra (sanskrit), Chobchini (Hindi, Punjabi), Kasbussini (Arabic), Chobchinae (Persian).

Family: *Smilacaceae* (formerly *Liliaceae*)

Species used: Numerous, the primary ones being: *S. glabra, S. officinalis, S. japicanga, S. febrifuga, S. regelii, S. aristolochiaefolia, S. ornata, S. zeylanica.*

Part used: The roots, generally six to eight feet long.

Collection and habitat: The roots can be collected at any time. Some 350 species of Smilax grow throughout the world's tropical and temperate regions, the primary species used medicinally being in China/Japan, South and Central America and the Caribbean. The plant itself is a brambled, woody vine that grows to 150 feet in length, often climbing high into the rainforest canopy.

Actions: Binds endotoxins in the blood (blood cleanser), immunomodulatory, antibacterial, antiparasitical, antiinflammatory, hepatoprotective, neuroprotective, enhances bioavailability of other herbs (and drugs), analgesic, antioxidant, antirheumatic, antiallergic, antiasthmatic, antimutagenic, antifungal, antifatigue.

Functions in Lyme disease: Smilax is a systemic herb with a wide range of actions in the body, many of which are specific for Lyme disease and its symptoms. Specifically: It lessens Herxheimer reactions from die-off of spirochetes (and Lyme coinfectious organisms) by its ability to bind endotoxins in the blood stream, it is antispirochetal, modulates immune response (lessening autoimmune reactions and stimulating specific immunity), enhances immune response to Lyme spirochetes, is antiinflammatory for arthritic symptoms, a neuroprotector for brain function (its constituents cross the blood/brain barrier), enhances cognitive function, reduces skin responses to Lyme disease (helpful in reducing and preventing symptoms of acrodermatitis chronica atrophicans which is common in European Lyme disease), enhances the actions of other herbs and drugs used in Lyme treatment, lessens fatigue, gives pain relief, and protects and enhances liver function.

Specific indications: Borrelia spp infections, with skin involvement, with arthritic inflammation, with Herxheimer reactions, with unresolved weakness, brain fog, confusion. Neuroborreliosis. Generally, any *Borrelia burgdorferi sensu lato* infection.

Plant chemistry: Extensive, primarily steroids and saponins. Steroids include: sarsapogenin, smilagenin, sitosterol, stigmasterol, and pollinastanol. Saponins include: sarsaponin, sarsasaponin, smilasaponin, and sarsaparilloside. A general list of plant chemicals also includes: cinchonin, isoseryl-s-methylcysteamine-sulfoxide, rutin, parillin, acetyl-parigenin, astilbin, beta-sitosterol, epsilon-sitosterol, sitosterol-d-glucoside, smilax saponins A-C, smiglaside A-E, smitilbin, caffeoyl-shikimic acids, dihydroquercetin, diosgenin, engeletin, eucryphin, euuryphin, ferulic acid, glucopyranosides, isoastilbin, isoengetitin, titogenin. There are a lot more, most of whose actions are unknown.

Medicinal uses of smilax: Smilax has been used for millennia among indigenous cultures for rheumatic complaints, skin problems (leprosy, psoriasis, dermatitis), low libido, and as a general tonic. Since the emergence of syphilis (and before antibiotics), it was used extensively for that condition throughout the world.

Ayurveda: Smilax has a long tradition of use in Ayurvedic, Siddha, and Unani practice throughout India for similar conditions: skin diseases, leprosy, kidney and bladder disease, paralysis, headache, convulsions, skin sores, rheumatic problems, epilepsy, dementia, syphilis, colic, pain.

Traditional Chinese medicine: In traditional Chinese medicine, smilax is used for turbid and painful urination, jaundice, recurrent ulcers or other skin lesions, pain in joints, liver and gall bladder problems, syphilis, leptospirosis, and tabes dorsalis (neurodegenerative syphilis).

Western botanic practice: Rather than moving into Europe from Asia as it could have done, smilax entered western practice in 1536 from European contact with the New World. It quickly found similar uses in European medical practice to those among the tribal groups where it grows and those in TCM and Ayurvedic practice: syphilis, rheumatic problems, blood purification, general tonic, gout, arthritis, fever, cough, scrofula, hypertension, digestive disorders, psoriasis and other skin disorders, and cancer. Its primary use has traditionally been for skin diseases, arthritis/rheumatic complaints, and syphilis.

Scientific: There was a flurry of interest in smilax studies (especially clinical trials) between 1935 and 1960, which then fell off as antibiotics and other pharmaceuticals came to dominate the market. There has been increased interest in the plant of late, which has again stimulated a number of *in vitro* and *in vivo* studies.

Smilax has been shown to be active against a number of parasitic, bacterial, and fungal organisms: leishmania, trypanosoma (sleeping sickness), treponema (syphilis), leptospira, *Clonorchia sinensis* (Chinese liver flukes), *Salmonella typhi, Salmonella enteritiditis, E. coli, Shigella dysenteriae, Shigella flexneri, Mycobacterium tuberculosis* (TB), *Mycobacterium leprae* (leprosy), and various dermatophytes (fungal skin infections).

Clinical trials using smilax in the treatment of leptospirosis in China found that prophylactic dosing with smilax decoctions (2-3 cups daily) significantly helped to prevent the onset of disease. In 2000 people tested, the incidence rate of leptospirosis compared with a control group was 1:5.58. In other words, in the untreated group there were five-and-a-half-times the number of leptospiral infections than in the treated group. Outcomes in the treatment of active leptospirosis improved with the use of the herb.

In one study, smilax was used in combination with other herbs (*Lonicera japonicus*, licorice, dandelion, *Dictamnus* spp) in the treatment of syphilis. (Smilax is considered to be the primary active herb in this formulation followed by lonicera). In 90% of those with acute syphilis and in 50% of those chronic syphilis, subsequent blood tests were negative for syphilitic organisms. In the treatment of tabes dorsalis (neurodegenerative syphilis), cerebrospinal fluid tested negative after use of the herb and mental and psychological parameters improved.

A clinical trial with smilax in the 1950s showed the herb more effective than sulfones in the treatment of leprosy. Another in 1942, reported in the *New England Journal of Medicine*, found that the herb significantly improved psoriasis. The study reported on the outcomes of a clinical trial with 92 people suffering from severe psoriasis. Sixty-two percent or 57 people experienced significant improvement in psoriatic lesions; 17 people cleared the condition completely, 18 showed no improvement. An earlier clinical study (1938) found the herb effective for both eczema and psoriasis.

Clinical studies have also found that the herb is effective for a variety of respiratory, allergic, and skin diseases. Specifically: bronchitis, bronchial asthma, allergic rhinitis, pollinosis, allergic conjunctivitis, atopic dermatitis, psoriasis, pustular psoriasis, exfoliative dermatitis, palmoplantaris keratosis, ichthyosis, pityriasis rubra pilaris.

Clinical studies in India have found that the herb is effective in treating cervical spondylosis, a degenerative condition of the spine.

Chinese clinical studies have found the herb useful in the treatment of type 2 diabetes. *In vivo* studies with mice have shown that the herb effectively lowers blood glucose levels.

A number of both clinical and *in vivo* studies have found the herb effective in increasing elimination of uric acid from the body in the treatment of gout.

In one clinical trial, the herb has been found effective in the treatment of liver disease. A randomized, double-blind, placebo study of a combined smilax/artichoke preparation was conducted with 60 people—53 male, seven female. All of the people suffered alcoholic hepatitis. The group was split randomly into two groups of 30 each. Dosage in the non-placebo group was three 420 mg capsules of the herb combination 3x daily for 30 days. The following changes were noted: Ascites: 72.38% reduction in treated group, 6.35% increase in treated group. Encephalopathy: 66.08% reduction in treated group, 12.24% increase in untreated group. Splenomegaly: 88.40% reduction in treated group, 11.54% increase in untreated group. Hepatomegaly: 93.33% reduction in treated group, 7.14% increase in untreated group. Weakness: 73.64% increase in strength in treated group, 7.41%

decrease in strength of the untreated group. Peripheral edema: Decreased in treated group by 48.21%, no change in placebo group. Hemorrhages: 100% decrease in treated group, 28.57% increase in placebo group. Anexoria: 76.98% decrease in treated group, decrease of 3.70% in placebo group. Palmar erythema: 26.67% reduction in treated group, no change in placebo group. Bilirubin: decrease in serum concentration in treated group by 38.95%, 5.68% increase in placebo group. APT: serum decrease in treated group by 25.91%, increase in untreated group by 11.69%. SGOT: decrease in treated group by 23.83%, increase in placebo group by 11.71%. Clotting time: decreased by 42% in treated group, increased in placebo by 6.60%.

Both *in vivo* and *in vitro* studies have found the herb effective in protecting the liver from damage by chemical assault, normalizing liver enzyme levels.

In vivo studies (in lab animals) have found smilax effective in autoimmune conditions, concomitant fibrosis or other tissue injury by, in part, selectively inhibiting activated T cells. Other *in vivo* studies have found the herb effective in the treatment of arthritis. It was found to affect both primary and secondary inflammation in adjunctive (drug-induced) arthritis by regulating cell-mediated immunity. The herb significantly inhibits swelling and lowers thymus and spleen weights.

In vivo and *in vitro* studies have found that the herb powerfully binds to endotoxins in the blood stream, reducing Herxheimer reactions from bacterial die-off. Endotoxins are toxins or substances, sometimes contained in the outer protein coat of the organism, sometimes inside their bodies, that are released when the organisms die.

Some of the more intriguing *in vivo* and *in vitro* studies have found several constituents of the herb, especially smilagenin, to be especially active in the brain where it shows marked inhibition and reversal of cognitive impairment. Two patents have been approved for use of the herb and its active constituents in the treatment of cognitive dysfunction conditions such as Alzheimer's disease and senile dementia. Extracts of the herb have been found to reverse the impacts of aging on rat cognition, returning them to the same level of performance as younger rats.

In vitro studies have shown activity against trypanosoma, leishmania, leptospira, TB, and a variety of other disease organisms. The herb's traditional use for bacterial dysentery among numerous peoples is supported by its *in vitro* actions against a number of pathogenic salmonella, shigella and *E. coli* bacteria.

Other *in vitro* studies have found the herb to possess antimutagenic, antitumor, anti-atherosclerosis activity, and to protect the male body from the impacts of anti-androgenic substances such as gossypol.

In general, for Lyme disease, the herb acts in the following areas: (1) it binds endotoxins, thus reducing Herxheimer reactions; (2) it is antispirochetal; (3) it is antiarthritic; (4) it acts in the brain to help reduce cognitive dysfunction and to protect from neurodegeneration; (5) normalizes autoimmune reactions; (6) helps in alleviating skin conditions attendant to Lyme infection; (7) enhances liver function; and (8) is broadly systemic in its actions including crossing the blood/brain barrier.

Dosage in Lyme disease: 425-500 mg capsules. One to three capsules 3-4x daily for 8-12 months. Begin at the lower dose and increase in increments every seven days as with the other herbs. Maintain highest dose for 60 days minimum. As Lyme symptoms reduce, the amount of herb can likewise be reduced, slowly, to a maintenance dose.

Contraindications: Large doses may cause intestinal upset.

Herb/drug interactions: Smilax can increase absorption of digitalis glycosides and bismuth. It increases elimination of hypnotic drugs.

Note: The bismuth/smilax interaction refers to large dose medical uses of bismuth.

CHAPTER FOUR

Expanding the Protocol:
An Herbal Repertory
for Lyme Disease

This expanded protocol is designed to allow a more comprehensive approach for those who do not intend to use antibiotics or if antibiotics have not previously been effective. It can be used along with antibiotics if desired.

The two most important things to consider in an expanded protocol are initiating a strong response at acute onset (also to be used for people who are experiencing severe symptoms) and support of the body's collagenous tissues. Lyme spirochetes love collagenous tissues and do considerable damage to them

IN THIS CHAPTER:
- Acute Onset of Lyme disease
- Herxheimer Reactions
- Collagenous tissue support
- Bell's Palsy and Ocularborreliosis
- Neurotoxin/neuroborreliosis
- Depression
- Lyme-specific Joint Pain/Arthritic Intervention
- General Arthritic Symptoms and Pain Relief
- Memory and Cognitive Dysfunction
- Angina and Heart Problems
- Eye Problems
- Muscle Twitches, Tingling/Crawling Sensation in Skin
- Swollen Lymph Nodes or Sluggish Lymph
- Muscle Weakness and Lack of Strength
- Candida Overgrowth
- Maintaining Intestinal Health on Antibiotics
- Headaches

whether in the knees, skin, heart, brain, or other organs.

The rest of the herbs and supplements in this section can be used to design a protocol for the particular symptom picture that a person with Lyme disease presents, thus making the protocol much more sophisticated in treating borrelia infections. The herbs and supplements discussed are listed under particular symptoms.

ACUTE ONSET OF LYME DISEASE
(And/or Severe Symptoms with Impairment)

ELEUTHERO, AKA SIBERIAN GINSENG (*Eleutherococcus senticosus, Acanthopanax senticosus*)

Common names: (English) eleuthero, siberian ginseng. (Chinese) ci-wu-jia.

Family: *Araliaceae*

Part used: The root.

Collection and Habitat: Siberian ginseng, a persistent, aggressive, shrub from three-to-fifteen feet in height, grows throughout parts of China, Russia, Korea, and even a bit in the northern islands of Japan. It is covered with spines and presents an aggressive, intimidating presence which has given rise to some of its common Russian names—Touch-me-not and Devil's shrub.

Due to its popularity as a medicinal, it is undergoing heavy planting in the United States and has begun to escape captivity. Soon it will be, like a number of important medicinals (among them Japanese knotweed), a naturalized, aggressive weed with qualities unknown to those it irritates.

The root is harvested in the fall, dried and processed for sale. When purchased, the root has generally already been cut-and-sifted or powdered to industry standards.

Adulteration of Chinese imports is a problem. North American-grown is generally more reliable.

Cultivation: From seeds.

Actions: Adaptogen, antistressor, immune tonic, immunpotentiator, immunoadjuvant, adrenal tonic, increases non-specific resistance against a number of pathogens, MAO inhibitor.

Functions in Lyme disease: Strongly initiates immune response to spirochete infection. Immune tonic and potentiator, adrenal tonic, antistressor, antidepressant, mental clarity stimulant, helps restore task endurance, enhances energy levels. By correcting adrenal function, it will help normalize thyroid function. The herb is an adaptogen, that is, a substance that increases nonspecific resistance to adverse influences.

Specific indications for use in Lyme infection: Chronic fatigue, mental fog and confusion, difficulty in overcoming the disease, low immune function.

About eleutherococcus: Although used in China for several thousand years, eleutherococcus (or Siberian ginseng as many people still prefer to call it) was used primarily by the Chinese for spasm. It was brought to prominence as an immune tonic and adaptogen by intensive Russian research in the latter half of the twentieth century (and has now traveled back to China as an adaptogenic herb). A number of clinical trials have shown significant immune-enhancing activity, including significant increases in immunocompetent cells, specifically T-lymphocytes (helper/inducers, cytotoxic, and natural killer cells). Tests of the herb have repeatedly shown that it increases the ability of human beings to withstand adverse conditions, increases mental alertness, and improves performance. People taking the herb consistently report fewer illnesses than those who do not take the herb. Part of its power is its ability to act as a tonic stimulant on the adrenal glands. It normalizes adrenal activity and moves adrenal action away from a cortisol/catabolic dynamic to a DHEA/anabolic orientation. Basically, this reduces stress and normalizes physiological functioning throughout the body.

In one Russian clinical trial, 2,100 healthy adults were given the herb and found to better handle stressful conditions. They showed increased ability to perform physical labor, withstand motion sickness, and work with speed and precision despite loud surroundings. Their ability to accurately proofread documents increased and they more readily adapted to diverse physical stresses—high altitudes, heat, and low-oxygen environments.

Another Russian study of 13,000 auto workers found that those who took the herb developed 40% fewer respiratory infections than normal for their group.

Other studies have found that the herb heightens mental alertness and improves concentration and boosts the transmission of nerve impulses in the brain.

Eleutherococcus senticosus and a related species *E. chiisanensis* have been found to be strongly antihepatotoxic and hepatoprotective *in vivo* against CCl4-induced hepatotoxicity. Additionally, Siberian ginseng was found to be a hepatoregenerator, significantly stimulating liver regeneration in animals with portions of their liver surgically removed.

As eleutherococcus is a MAO inhibitor it is also useful in depression, a condition that often accompanies a severely depleted immune system, chronic fatigue-like diseases, and Lyme infection.

Russian Dosages: Most of the Russian studies were conducted using a 1:1 tincture using 30%-33% alcohol. The dosage ranged from 2-20 milliliters per day (the smaller dose is about one-half teaspoon of tincture). This means people were taking from one-sixteenth to two-thirds of an ounce (and in some instances up to one and one-half ounces) of tincture per day. At an average cost of seven to twelve dollars per ounce of tincture this can be prohibitively expensive at the upper dosage ranges.

The Russians generally dosed 2-16 ml, 1-3x day for 60 days with a two to three week rest period in between. Russian researchers, at these kinds of dosages, saw responses within a few days or even hours of administration. Some of the American companies that utilize the Russian approach for tincturing also like to standardize their formulas for specific eleutheroside content as well.

Dosage in Lyme disease: *Please read carefully.* In acute onset Lyme disease (or Lyme disease with severe symptoms) the stronger Russian formulation is the only type of tincture that should be used. I suggest the product made by Herb Pharm, which is the only company I know of that actually exceeds the Russian specifications. Their formula is a 2:1 rather than a 1:1 (i.e., two parts herb to one part liquid).

For the first 30-60 days: one teaspoon 3x daily, the last dose occurring by 4:00 pm. This can be increased if necessary.

Discontinue the herb for two weeks.

Then repeat if necessary.

If symptoms decrease after using the Russian formulation and immune function seems better, the type of formulation used can change to either an encapsulated form or a 1:5 alcohol/water tincture (one part herb to five parts liquid). Both these formulations are weaker than the Russian approach.

As an encapsulated form, I suggest a 450 mg capsule of a formulation standardized to 0.8% eleutherosides B&E. I suggest Nature's Way, which contains 250 mg of standardized extract and 200 mg of the whole herb. Two capsules 4x daily for the 8-12 months of treatment.

Note: If symptoms and overall health are better on the extract than the capsules, or if the presenting symptoms are severe, then the extract may be a better choice for continual use. Continue the tincture 30-60 days on, 2-3 weeks off, 30-60 days on, and so on.

Other preparations and dosages: I have generally used, and prefer in conditions other than Lyme disease or severe chronic fatigue, a weaker tincture, as do many American herbalists and herbal companies: 1:5, 60% alcohol, full dropper (one-third teaspoon) of the tincture 1-3x day for up to a year. In my experience this dosage and pattern of use is less stimulating to the system and the long term effects are better. The body gradually uses the herb to build itself up over time, the herb acting more as a long-term tonic and rejuvinative than an active stimulant. With this type of tincture it is not necessary to stop every one to two months, nor have I seen any of the side effects that can occur with the stronger Russian formula.

In my clinical experience, this weaker, American tincture takes six months to become really effective and should be used at least that long, a year is better. It is great for long-term, chronic conditions that are not resolving. It acts as a very deep tonic to the system. However, in acute conditions such as acute-onset Lyme disease or severe chronic fatigue, the stronger Russian formulation is essential. Once the acute condition resolves, you can move to the weaker 1:5 formulation.

The Chinese, much less given to tincturing anyway, use 4.5-27 grams, often as a decoction or powder.

Side effects and contraindications: Insomnia and hyperactivity can occur with use of the stronger Russian formulation, especially when taken in large doses, with caffeine, or late in the afternoon or evening.

Eleutherococcus is, in general, completely nontoxic and the Russians have reported the use of exceptionally large doses for up to 20 years with no adverse reactions. It is especially indicated for people with pale, unhealthy skin, lassitude, and depression.

For almost all people no side effects have been noted. A very small number of people have experienced transient diarrhea. The Russian formulation may temporarily increase blood pressure in some people. This tends to drop to normal within a few weeks. Caution should be exercised for people with very high blood pressure especially if combined with other hypertensives such as licorice. With extreme overuse—tension and insomnia.

HERXHEIMER REACTIONS

Smilax can be useful during Lyme infection, especially for Herxheimer reactions where it finds its most potent use. It is one of the few herbs that will strongly bind endotoxins and the byproducts from bacterial die-off.

COLLAGENOUS TISSUE SUPPORT

Lyme spirochetes cause a great deal of destruction to collagenous tissues throughout the body. The core protocol will help with this, but if you are suffering severe side effects of the disease or suspect that its course might be severe, you should consider initiating a regimen specifically designed to support the collagenous structures in the body. The following supplements are the most powerful for doing so.

Vitamin C

The vitamin C-dependant enzyme, pro-lyl hydroxylase, is the catalyst that enables collagen to form. Without vitamin C, prolyl hydroxylase cannot maintain activity, collagen cannot form fibers properly and bones, cartilage and skin cannot heal efficiently.

During collagen synthesis, vitamin C acts as an essential co-enzyme. For this reason, collagen is usually high in vitamin-C content and deficiencies have been found to reduce cartilage repair and synthesis processes.

If you are suffering collagen breakdown from Lyme, vitamin C is essential to support the body's creation of new collagen tissues.

Dosage: 1,000-3,000 mg daily.

> **COLLAGENOUS TISSUE PROTOCOL**
>
> *Please read contraindications carefully.*
>
> Pregnenolone: 50-200 mg daily
>
> Zinc picolinate with copper: 20-30 mg daily
>
> Silicon (as stabilized orthosilicic acid): 6-20 drops daily
>
> DHEA: 15-200 mg daily
>
> Alpha Lipoc Acid: 600 mg daily
>
> Selenium: 200 mcg daily
>
> Glucosamine sulfate: 500 mg 3x day
>
> Vitamin B complex: daily, should include B-5, B-6, B-12, and folic acid)
>
> Vitamin C: 1,000-3,000 mg daily.
>
> Vitamin E: 400-800 IU daily.

Note: I prefer a powdered, effervescent form of vitamin C (see resource section for sources).

Side effects: Vitamin C at larger doses will cause flatulence and loose stools, upset stomach, or diarrhea. If you experience these symptoms, reduce the dose and begin to work up to higher doses as your body adjusts. Breaking up the dose you take into two or three doses will often allow a two-to-three times increase in the amount you can take before side effects occur. Vitamin C is sometimes prescribed t.b.t—to bowel tolerance—meaning you take it until side effects occur.

Note: Many of the herbs and medications used to treat Lyme infections can cause constipation. Vitamin C is the best supplement to use to normalize bowel flow if this occurs. It corrects the constipation while adding a substance exceptionally useful to the body during Lyme infection.

Zinc picolinate with copper

Both zinc and copper have been found to be essential for proper collagen formation. Copper is a critical cofactor in collagen production and, as well, is essential for the maintenance of collagen status in the arterial walls. Low levels of both zinc and copper have been found in people suffering collagenous diseases. Because zinc picolinate with copper is so essential in treating Lyme neurotoxins and collagen support, it should be added to all Lyme protocols.

Dosage: 20-30mg daily

Silicon

Silicon is required for the synthesis of proline and hydroxyproline, both essential in cartilage formation and maintenance. It is also required for the synthesis of glycocaminoglycans where it acts as a cross-linking agent. It is very active in the heart's collagenous tissues. Low levels of silicon have been found in people suffering various forms of heart disease. Silicon is also involved in myelin production and supplementation will help protect and restore damaged myelin sheaths during Lyme infection of the CNS.

Silicon is an essential supplement for Lyme borreliosis.

Dosage: 6-20 drops daily in one-quarter cup water of a stabilized orthosilicic acid supplement. BioSil is one possible brand of many.

Glucosamine Sulfate (GS)

Glucosamine, naturally produced by the body, is used to stimulate the body's production of glycosaminoglycans. These are the compounds that give cartilage its rubber-like nature. As people age, they tend to produce less GS, which results in poorer cartilage formation. This becomes especially problematic in joints that receive a lot of wear and tear: hips, knees, hands, neck, and back. The great strength of GS is that it promotes the regeneration and replacement of cartilage. A number of controlled, double-blind trials (with up to 1,500 people at a time) have been conducted and GS has been found to be highly effective in the treatment of osteoarthritis. While those in the trials who were taking strong analgesics experienced relief more quickly, those who were taking GS pulled ahead after four weeks. The longer GS was taken, the better the results. The trial results indicated that GS appears to address the underlying symptoms and actually cure the condition, something pain medications do not do. Those taking the supplement were found, after four weeks, to have less pain, better mobility, less stiffness, and an expanded sense of well being. Ninety-five percent of those taking GS report benefit. Normally, GS needs to be taken at least four weeks to show benefit; the longer it is taken, the longer benefits last after ceasing use.

Dosage: 500 mg 3x day

COMMENT: About Chondroitin Sulfate: Although chondroitin sulfate (CS) has been touted for this same use, increasingly, evidence indicates it is not very effective. Some research has shown that while GS absorption into the body is generally higher than 90%, CS is often 13% or less. A majority of practitioners now recommend GS over CS for that reason.

Pregnenolone

Pregnenolone was one of the earliest medical treatments for both osteo- and rheumatoid arthritis and was commonly prescribed by physicians in the 1950s. After the arrival of synthetic cortisones, the exploration into pregnenolone's effectiveness unfortunately ceased. Pregnenolone has shown specific beneficial activity for a wide range of connective tissue disorders: ankolysing spondylitis, systemic lupus, osteo- and rheumatoid arthritis, and scleroderma. All these diseases are concerned with improper collagen formation, deterioration, or inflammation.

Numerous studies in the 1950s commonly found that people who take pregnenolone can experience significant alleviation of arthritic symptoms, generally less pain, more mobility, and less stiffness. In the five studies I have reviewed, about one-third of the people experienced a near complete remission of symptoms, one third had marked improvement, and one third showed no benefit. Improvement was generally seen within sixty days. The longer pregnenolone was taken in the studies, the longer benefits lasted after supplementation ceased. Pregnenolone exerts direct effects on the body's capillaries, skin, collagen formation, and mucous membranes. In treatment of scleroderma (a hardening of the skin), pregnenolone was found to soften the skin, increasing elasticity and texture. Pregnenolone also tends to produce an increased sense of well being, more energy, better appetite, and enhanced memory.

In Lyme disease, it is specifically helpful for supporting collagen in skin, joints, and reducing arthritic and skin symptoms.

Dosage: 50-500 mg daily

Side effects and contraindications: At higher doses pregnenolone can cause agitation and overstimulation. The best average dosing for arthritic conditions seems to be 100-200 mg daily.

DHEA (Dehydroepiandrosterone)

In clinical trials with people suffering lupus (a collagen, connective tissue disease), 200 mg daily of DHEA was found to decrease symptoms, pain, progression of the disease, and need for corticosteroids. There were far fewer flareups in those taking DHEA than in the placebo group. DHEA has also been found to be especially low in people with rheumatoid arthritis (RA). Using the supplement has been found to help with symptoms of RA just as it has with lupus.

Dosage: Men 50-200 mg daily; women 15-25 mg daily.

Side effects and contraindications: There is slight potential for women to experience androgenation from intake of high DHEA levels. Higher dosage levels are contraindicated for adolescent males.

Alpha Lipoc Acid

Alpha lipoic acid (ALA) is a powerful antioxidant, chelation agent, radioprotective agent, enzymatic catalyst, glutathione production stimulant, normalizer of blood sugar levels, neurotonic, and antiviral. It is exceptionally potent as a protector and regenerator of liver tissue. It has also been found to enhance energy, increase memory and mental clarity, and reduce joint inflammation. For all these reasons it is worthwhile to consider using it in Lyme disease.

ALA was isolated from liver tissue in 1951. It turns out that human cells, especially in the liver, naturally produce ALA, although as we grow older we make less and less of it. In general, ALA does two things. It acts as a helper, a coenzyme, to our body's cells in utilizing energy (glucose). It also is one of the most powerful antioxidants known, helping prevent damage to cells at the genetic level. Antioxidants protect our bodies from the effects of reactive oxygen species (ROS), including free radicals. Vitamin C, a well-known antioxidant, is very large and can only protect the cells from the outside. Because ALA is so small, it can pass inside the cells and protect both the inside and outside from the oxidative stress effects of free radicals. People with RA have been found to consistently have lower levels of antioxidants in their bodies.

This antioxidant action of glutathione as well in Lyme disease. Glutathione, ALA, and vitamin C all will help remove endotoxins from Lyme spirochetes from the system, and potentiate the immune response to the bacteria and its toxins.

Glutathione is also exceptionally low in autoimmune arthritic conditions like rheumatoid arthritis. Many people who have increased their glutathione levels through the use of ALA or other glutathione enhancers, have found that as body levels of glutathione (and selenium) rise their symptoms disappear. For this reason, it makes sense to use ALA (or another glutathione enhancer such as N-acetyl cysteine) if you have an autoimmune-type arthritis. Glutathione, as well, reduces the production of inflammatory prostaglandins and leukotrienes, which is one reason ALA has been found to be directly effective in joint inflammation.

ALA is strongly antiviral both directly and indirectly by increasing glutathione levels. In a number of studies, German researchers have found ALA to be effective in the treatment of AIDS patients. After fourteen days of use, they found that plasma ascorbate and glutathione levels both increased. The higher the level of glutathione, the lower the level of HIV. While ALA is itself directly antiviral against a number of viruses, glutathione is even more effective. Emerging research indicates that glutathione acts as a powerful antiviral in the body and is produced, in part, for that reason. It is highly synergistic with selenium (its mineral cofactor) in carrying out antiviral actions.

Dosage: 600 mg daily.

Caution: Diabetics should use only after review with their physician. ALA strongly affects blood sugar levels and will affect medical protocols. N-acetyl cysteine (NAC) is an effective substitute for ALA, 1200 mg daily.

Selenium

Selenium is the cofactor of glutathione; it must be present for glutathione to be created in the body. It has also been found to be a powerful antiviral.

It is now known that a significant number of viruses (HIV, Epstein-barr, influenza, and hepatitis C, for example) have developed strategies to reduce levels of the body's selenium. As selenium levels fall, the natural antiviral actions of the body's selenium and glutathione decrease, allowing viral blooms to occur. People with rheumatoid arthritis (RA) generally have low levels of selenium. One study has shown that supplementation with selenium and vitamin E relieved symptoms of RA.
Dosage: 200 mcg (micrograms) daily.

Vitamin B complex

Low vitamin B-5 (pantothenic acid) levels have been found to cause a failure of healthy cartilage growth. For some people with osteoarthritis, as little as 12.5 mg of B-5 daily have significantly reduced symptoms. A good vitamin B complex should be added that contains at least this much B-5.
Dosage: 1-2 tablets daily.

Vitamin E

Because vitamin E potentiates both vitamin C and selenium in cartilage tissue, it is important to include. An even more important reason to include vitamin E is that it stimulates CD57 white blood cells, the same ones that cat's claw stimulates. This stimulation is important as chronic Lyme disease generally presents with low CD57 counts.
Dosage: 400-800 IU daily.

BELL'S PALSY
AND OCULARBORRELIOSIS

Bell's palsy is more accurately known as partial facial paralysis. Lyme infections can affect the nerve in the face (seventh cranial nerve) that controls facial movements: inflammation from spirochetal infection sets in, the nerve swells, it compresses against the bone, and one side (usually) of the face freezes in place. Demyelination of the nerve (basically, destruction of the nerve sheath) can also cause the problem. Both of these initiating conditions can be caused by Lyme spirochetes. Most Bell's palsy in Lyme infections occur in children who experience a tick bite on the neck, near the site of the nerve. Up to one-fourth of new Bell's palsy occurrences are from Lyme infection.

Treatment usually involves alleviating the source of infection or inflammation, which then reduces the swelling and the condition improves. Antibiotics are almost always effective for this symptom of Lyme infection. The condition may take several weeks to reverse, even with antibiotics. Two closely related plants—*Stephania tetrandra* and *Stephania cepharantha*—have been found effective. (Acupuncture may also be of use in recalcitrant cases.) These two stephanias possess very similar actions and may be used interchangeably (see the plant description for subtleties). (There are a number of other stephanias that are used medicinally as well but they should not be substituted; they are not interchangeable.) In general, *S. cepharantha* may be slightly better for neural inflammations and *S. tetrandra* for ocular problems in the treatment of Lyme borreliosis.

Stephania species may be able to play a larger role in Lyme borreliosis in that the plants are specific for nerve inflammations, acting as neuroprotectors in the brain from inflammatory conditions. They are also specific for arthritic inflammations that have an autoimmune dynamic such as rheumatoid arthritis. They have angiogenesis-modulating actions, and exhibit a number of positive cardiovascular actions—helping with arrhythmia, infarction, coronary flow, and heart rate. These *Stephania* species, especially *S. tetrandra*, are specific for Lyme-initiated eye inflammations. In fact, the whole range of ocular manifestations of Lyme can be successfully treated with the herb. The herbs also interfere with cellular adhesion and chemotaxis and protect endothelial cells. There is the potential that the herbs can interfere with the chemotactic and cellular adhesion dynamics of Lyme borrelia. And finally, the herbs have been found to potentiate the actions of antibiotics and other pharmaceuticals in the treatment of cancers and various diseases such as malaria. Drugs inactivated by the cancers or microbes through various resistance mechanisms are potently effective when readministered with either of these two species. Early findings also indicate that the stephanias potentiate the actions of herbs as well.

The broad range of actions of these herbs, corresponding to many Lyme conditions, and the unusual nature of their underlying actions suggest that they are potentially significant herbs for use in the treatment of Lyme borreliosis. Regrettably, they are somewhat difficult to obtain, especially *S. cepharantha*. Bulk quantities of *S. tetrandra* can be ordered from a few Chinese medicine importers and generally must be prepared for use as capsules, tinctures, decoctions, or infusions (see Resources).

The difficulty in obtaining a reliable supply of the herb is the reason that stephania root is not included in the core protocol.

STEPHANIA ROOT (*Stephania tetrandra, S. cepharantha*)

Common names: *S. tetrandra* and *S. cepharantha* are the main species used medicinally (at least for our purposes). For both: Stephania root in English and Hang-fang-ji in China (Pinyin). However distinctions are made with those that know these closely-related *Stephania* plants. *Stephania tetrandrae*: Fourstamen stephania root (English), (Pinyin) Hang-fang-ji or baimuxiang, (Japanese) kanboi, (Korean) hang-banggi. *Stephania cepharantha*: Oriental stephania root (English), (Pinyin) baiyaozi, (Japanese) Haku-yaku-shi. There are a number of other species that are also used (but are not interchangeable with these two): *Stephania dielsiana*: Diels stephania root (English), (Pinyin) xuesanshu. *Stephania japonica*: Japanese stephania root (English). (Pinyin) qianjinteng. *Stephania epigaea*: Epigeal Stephania root (English), (Pinyin) diburong. *Stephania longa*: Long stephania root (English), (Pinyin) fenjidu. Japonica is probably the most common of these other species.

Family: Menispermiaceae

Part Used: The root and rootlets, sometimes the vine.

Collection and Habitat: This species likes the jungle and warm climates. It is native to Asia and is commonly found in Japan, China, Taiwan, Vietnam, Australia and so on. Various species are used by indigenous peoples throughout the region. *S. tetrandra* is native to China where most of the research on it has occurred. *S. cepharantha* is common in Japan where most of its research has occurred. *S. tetrandra* is grown commercially for medicinal use in China in the regions of Zhejiang, Anhui, Jiangxi, and Hubei.

The plants are unusual. The primary root looks much like a rock or boulder and grows on top of the ground. Irregularly spaced rootlets one-to-three inches or more in diameter, occasionally on the side but primarily underneath, extend from this into the ground. The plants may take as long as 150 years to reach maturity. The globular-shaped, rock-like root, at that point, may be as much as three feet in diameter and weigh up to 200 pounds. At fifty years of age, they are the size of a basketball and weigh about 40 pounds.

Local peoples sometimes refer to the plant as a "mountain turtle" as its bark resembles a turtle shell. The plant extends a vine covered with heart-shaped leaves into the overstory, using trees for support. The vine thickens and is often harvested for medicine instead of the root. It is these vines and rootlets that have often (in the past) been confused, when dried and sliced, with an aristolochia species with a similar Chinese name (see Side Effects). The root is, however, considered to be better as a medicinal than the vines.

The plant flowers May-June, fruits July-September. Melon-sized roots are often harvested for use, sliced and dried. They should be a light tan in color. They are usually harvested in the fall.

Cultivation: From seeds or a transplanted root the size of a cherry.

Actions: Antiarthritic, anti-inflammatory, antiedema, calcium-channel blocker, vasodilator, antifibrotic, analgesic, smooth muscle relaxant,

Antiparasitic, antipyretic, antitumor, antibacterial, diuretic, drug-synergist, angiogenesis modulator, sedative, antiasthmatic, ascites.

Constituents: Slightly different for both. *S. tetrandra:* Tetrandrine, fangchinoline, menisine, menisidine, cyclanoline, stephanthrine, oxo-fangchinoline, 2-N-methyltetrandrine, fanchinin, isotetrandrine, cyclanoline, demethyltetrandrine, handfangchins, stearic-acid-glyc-erides. *S. cepharantha:* cepharanthine, tetrandrine, isotetrandrine, cycleanine, berbamine, homoaromoline, cephalamine, cepharanoline, trilobine.

Functions in Lyme infection: For neural and arthritic inflammations, ocularborreliosis, edema, myalgias, endothelial protection, and as an immunomodulator.

Specific indications: Bell's palsy, ocular involvement during Lyme infection (ocularborreliosis—uveitis, conjunctivitis, etc), Lyme arthritis with edema in the knee (or other joint), neuroborreliosis, antibiotic-resistant Lyme arthritis, late stage Lyme infections of nervous system, joints, and skin.

Note: Caution should be exercised in the use of this herb for Lyme carditis.

About stephania: *Stephania* species have a long history of use in China and Japan for a number of conditions; it is virtually unknown in the west.

Ayurveda: Unknown, although two other stephania species are used, primarily for diarrhea, dyspepsia, and urinary problems.

Traditional Chinese medicine: *S. tetrandra* has been used for millennia in China. Its uses correspond to those actions listed above: pain, edema (especially in lower parts of the body), ascites, abdominal distention, fever, red, hot, swollen and painful joints.

Western botanic practice: Unknown in the past and relatively unknown now, it is very rarely used among western practitioners.

Scientific: Nearly all of the research on these plants is occurring in Asia, primarily China and Japan, and comes out of their long history of plant medicines and healing.

The three constituents most tested for pharmacological actions from these two plants are tetrandrine, cepharanthine, and berbamine.

Tetrandrine and cepharanthine are considered the most potent. Their molecular structures are very similar; both are bisbenzylisoquinoline alkaloids (as is berbamine). Their pharmacological actions are very similar as well; they are considered to have comparable immunopharmacology. Most research on *S. tetrandra* constituents is occurring in China, *S. cepharantha* research is mostly in Japan. Medline lists 458 studies on tetrandrine and 168 on various *Stephania* species, primarily *S. tetrandra*. Cepharanthin(e) shows 187 Medline citations.

The Japanese have put together a proprietary herbal formulation—basically a root extract—called cepharanthin that is standardized around five of the alkaloids from *S. cepharnatha*: cepharanthine, berbamine, homoaromoline, cepharanoline, and cycleanine. These make up 90% of the formulation's content, another 46 compounds make up the remaining 10%. The constituents are highly bioavaiable when taken orally. It is available in liquid and oral form and is used in Japan for the treatment of chronic inflammatory diseases, radiation-induced leukopenia, bronchial asthma, and alopecia areata. This formulation is not yet available in Europe or the U.S.

Stephania, as an herb, is becoming known in the west primarily for the treatment of baldness (why am I not surprised?). In a number of studies, it has shown better effects than the pharmaceuticals used for that condition.

Lyme borrelia stimulate the production of interleukin-1-beta (IL-1b) and to a lesser extent, IL-alpha, tumor necrosis factor-alpha (TNF-a), IL-6, and IL-8 in a number of locations in the body including the brain and at joint locations. Stephania root is specific for reducing these particular cytokines (and chemokine). The plant alkaloids cross the blood/brain barrier and act powerfully in reducing inflammation in the brain. The anti-inflammatory effect of stephania is considered to be corticosteroid-like in its effectiveness. It is especially effective for reducing NF-kB and IL-6 levels in the brain during neuroborreliosis.

Antibiotic-resistant Lyme arthritis has been connected to the expression of CD3-generated HLA-DR alleles. Stephania specifically modulates HLA-DR expression (as well as CD23 and CD25) making it specific in the treatment of resistant Lyme arthritis.

Tetrandrine (Tet) has been found to inhibit neutrophil and monocyte adhesion. Clinical trials have found it effective in the treatment of silicosis, where it retards and even reverses silicosis lesions. Lymphoproliferative responses are markedly reduced, neutrophil random movement, chemotaxis, and phagocytosis are significantly suppressed. Tet inhibits prostaglandin and TNF-alpha generation by monocytes. Tet (and *S. tetrandra*) specifically protect endothelial cells from endotoxin damage and inhibits inflammation and reduces vascular permeability. The herb tends to reduce overly exuberant immune responses by certain lymphocyte subsets while allowing CD4 levels to remain high.

It has been found to reduce edema and increased vascular permeability and plasma extravasation in Bell's palsy. The herb and constituent decrease the significantly increased levels of IL-6, IL-8, and TNF-alpha that occur during Bell's palsy.

It is a powerful free-radical scavenger and its constituents fangochinoline and tetrandrine, are powerful neuroprotectors against such things as H2O2 (hydrogen peroxide). The constituents inhibit H2O2-induced neuronal cell death, inhibit the elevation of glutamate and cytosolic free Ca2+ concentration, and the generation of reactive oxygen species (ROS).

The herb and its constituents are powerful calcium-channel blockers, although by mechanisms previously unknown and very different than those of pharmaceuticals. They have been found effective in the treatment of hypertension, cardiac diseases, asthma and other inflammatory pulmonary diseases. Tet directly blocks both T-type and L-type calcium current in ventricular cells and vascular smooth muscle cells. It has been found effective in the treatment of arrythmia, angina, and myocardial infarction. Diastolic amplitude, total apexcardiographic relaxation index, diastolic amplitude time index all improved significantly with Tet (better than verapamil).

Both the herb and tetrandrine are specific for eye conditions associated with Lyme infection. The herb has generated interest because of its effectiveness for treating neovascularization of the retinal capillary (retinopathy) in diabetes. Tet has been determined to be the primary active constituent. Use of the herb or Tet blocks neovascularization in streptozotocin-induced diabetic rats in both the retinal and choroidal capillaries. Other *in vivo* studies found that Tet inhibited choroidal and air-pouch granuloma angiogenesis. Tet was found to inhibit allergin-stimulated conjunctivitis, significantly reducing conjunctival eosinophil infiltration and the number of intact and degranulating mast cells. It inhibited IL-1b and TNF-alpha as well. It was found to be as effective as antiallergenic drugs. Tet has been found to be specific for uveitis in a number of *in vivo* studies.

Tet is a potent anti-inflammatory agent—more so than the corticosteroid prednisolone—in treating various retinopathies resulting from ocular ischemia and or inflammation.

Tet has been found to be a potent inhibitor of multi-drug resistance in the treatment of cancers and malaria. Malarial parasites resistant to chloroquine were killed when retreated with Tet and chloroquine together. Similar impacts have been found with a number of multi-drug-resistant cancers.

These kinds of actions have been found in the closely related compound, cepharanthine, and with the proprietary Japanese combination cepharanthin. Cepharanthin is fifty times more potent than verapamil, a pharmaceutical resistance modulator and three times more potent than any of the five individual alkaloids that make up the combination.

Cepharanthine has also been found to downregulate MMP-9, NF-kB, PKC, IL-1b, IL-6, IL-8, and TNF-alpha and to stabilize mast cells, protect membranes from permeability enhancement, scavenge ROS, block histamine release, and to be strongly antifibrotic. It also possesses antimicrobial actions against TB, leprosy, and malaria (mild). It directly inhibits cancer cell proliferation.

These two stephania species are specific for Lyme infection and many of its effects. They should definitely be considered for use in late-stage Lyme arthritis as a major component of any herbal treatment regimen, Bell's palsy that will not correct with antibiotics, and ocular manifestations of Lyme infection.

Dosage for Lyme Infection: The herb powders easily and can be encapsulated, tinctured, or heated with water as an infusion or decoction. Tincture the herb (either herb individually, or a combination of the two stephania species, equal parts) in a 1:5, 65% alcohol/water solution. If encapsulating the herb, use one-to-four "00" capsules, 3-4x daily beginning at the lowest dose and working up (as with the core protocol). In Bell's palsy, the most efficient form of the herb is the tincture or decoction.

Bell's Palsy: one teaspoon 3x daily of the tincture

Neuroborreliosis: one half teaspoon 3x daily of the tincture

Lyme Arthritis: one half teaspoon 3x daily of the tincture

Ocularborreliosis: one half teaspoon 3x daily of the tincture, eye wash with the decoction daily

In Chinese medicine, 3-9 grams of the whole herb are taken daily or 5-10 grams slow-boiled (simmered) in one-half to one quart of water (decoction) for 60 minutes and consumed daily. The decoction can be used topically for eye inflammations as well as taken internally. It should be allowed to cool before application.

The herb is moderately mucilaginous when cooked, and will clump together in a glue-like mass in the pan as it simmers. The resulting liquid will be somewhat thickened, like a thinnish gruel. It is moderately bitter, although nothing like andrographis.

If ever available in the west, the use of the Japanese formulation, cepharanthin, should be explored in the treatment of Lyme borreliosis as a supportive adjunct to antibiotic therapies.

Other Products: There are a number of stephania combination formulas on the market, e.g. stephania/clematis, stephania/astragalus. Product labels should be carefully read to make sure that they do actually contain *Stephania tetrandra* or equivalent. There may be as many as 10 herbs in these formulations and you should check the amount of stephania before taking them. Clematis/stephania may be a good combination for neuroborreliosis although I do not know of anyone who has tried it for the condition. It is specific for nerve damage, pain, etc.

Side Effects: Constipation. Calcium channel blockers cause constipation in about half the people using them. If this occurs the herb should be taken with vitamin C, dosed to bowel tolerance.

No other side effects have been reported. **However**, the plant has sometimes been confused with an aristolochia species, *Aristolochia fangchi*, whose Chinese name is similar—guang fang ji. That aristolochia species was sent, instead of stephania root, for instance, to a Belgian weight-loss clinic that used it in treatment. A number of incidents of nephropathy with renal failure occurred among the patients at the clinic and stephania root was blamed. Examination, however, showed that stephania was not present, but rather *Aristolochia fangchi*. That particular plant contains aristolochic acid as a constituent, which can be a potent kidney toxin *when the plant is tinctured*: in water, it is relatively benevolent. Aristolochic acid-related nephropathy is a common side effect from improper use of aristolochic acid-containing plants.

Product safety: After those problems with adulterants, all *Stephania spp.* herbal manufacturers and importers began testing the identity of the herb for accuracy prior to sale. Plum Flower Brand, which is the primary source available in the U.S., is stringently tested prior to sale.

Contraindications: Atrioventricular block. The constituents of these plants, especially tetrandrine, are potent calcium-channel blockers although their mechanism of action is decidedly unusual. They do not block through the same mechanisms of action as pharmaceuticals and are considered to be a new class of calcium-channel blocker. However, calcium-channel blockers are contraindicated in atrioventricular block. There is no evidence that these plants would produce poor outcomes in AV block, but caution should be exercised in its use where AV block is present during Lyme infection.

Herb/drug interactions: Not to be used with people taking pharmaceutical calcium-channel blockers or beta-blocker drugs. Not for use with people taking digoxin. Not for use with people on anti-arrhythmic medications. Not to be used with people who are severely hypotensive.

Drug/herb synergist. May potentiate the action of pharmaceuticals and other herbs. The plant and its constituents, tetrandrine and cepharathine, have generated interest because they have shown remarkable activity in potentiating the activity of pharmaceuticals— Tetrandrine in the treatment of multiple-drug-resistant cancers of various types (as well as malaria) and cepharanthin and cepharanthine with malaria.

LYME NEUROTOXIN/NEUROBORRELIOSIS INTERVENTION

Quinolinic acid, produced in the brain and CSF during Lyme infection, is a potent neurotoxin. Many of the effects of QUIN, as it is colloquially known, can be ameliorated or prevented by the use of some easy-to-find supplements. These will work synergistically with many of the herbs in the core protocol to increase antioxidant activity in the brain and protect the CNS from damage. *Polygonum cuspidatum* is especially synergistic with these supplements.

Resveratrol (*Polygonum cuspidatum*)

Polygonum cuspidatum (through its constituent, resveratrol) will help considerably with the neurological impacts of quinolinic acid through two mechanisms. First, resveratrol is a potent antioxidant. It potentiates the actions of other antioxidants, both naturally occurring and ingested, reduces oxidative stress, and protects against reactive oxygen species (ROS) impacts on the brain. Second, resveratrol's molecular structure is very similar to diethylstilbestrol, a synthetic estrogen. Studies have found that resveratrol acts much like the natural estrogen estradiol in the body (without producing many of estradiol's negative side effects). Estradiol has been found to reduce QUIN insults to the brain *in vivo*. QUIN production is stimulated by interferon-gamma (IFN-g) production and resveratrol down-regulates IFN-g-medi-

> **LYME NEUROTOXIN PROTOCOL**
>
> Resveratrol (core protocol)
>
> Selenium, 200 mcg daily
>
> Zinc picolinate with copper, 20-30 mg daily
>
> Melatonin, 1-3 mg daily

ated effects including QUIN and neopterin production. See core protocol listing for more on this plant and resveratrol.

Selenium

Selenium has been tested *in vivo* and *in vitro* and found to be specifically active in protecting the central nervous system against different markers of QUIN-induced neurotoxicity. Selenium is, however, only partially protective, showing protection in specific areas of the brain but not all those affected by QUIN. It decreases oxidative impacts in synaptosomes in the striatum and hippocampus but not in the cortex, and significantly attenuates striatal GABA depletion and the ratio of neuronal damage.

Dosage: 200-400 mcg (micrograms) daily

Cautions: 400 mcg is the highest dose that should be used, as side effects begin to occur beyond this dose range. The best average daily dose in Lyme disease is 200 mcg.

Side effects: (at high dosages.) Nausea, vomiting, emotional instability. Through a number of mechanisms selenium may deplete the body's levels of zinc and copper. It should be taken with a zinc/copper supplement.

Zinc Picolinate with Copper

Studies have found that while zinc ions can possess neurotoxic effects under some circumstances, zinc itself is able to prevent hippocampal neuronal damage from QUIN. Zinc supplementation has been found to be neuroprotective against the neurotoxicity of excitotoxins such as QUIN.

Copper blocks the neurotoxicity of QUIN as well. *In vivo* studies found that copper counteracted the neurotoxic activity of QUIN. It reduced striatal GABA depletion and blocked oxidative injury to neurons. The researchers commented that "at low doses, copper exerts a protective effect on *in vivo* QUIN neurotoxicity."

Both copper and zinc supplementation increase the actions of the copper/zinc-dependent superoxide dismutase, a potent ROS scavenger.

Picolinic acid also blocks the neurotoxic effects of QUIN *in vivo*. Specifically, it blocks the cholinergic neurotoxicity induced by QUIN in the frontoparietal cortex. Choline acetyl-transferase activity remained unaffected by QUIN when PA was present.

Picolinic acid is a natural derivative of the amino acid tryptophan. Metals such as zinc are often bound to picolinic acid to aid absorption. And often, with zinc supplementation, copper is also added. A common combination is 30 mg zinc picolinate with 2 mg copper. The combination zinc picolinate with copper is specific for the kinds of neurotoxicity produced by QUIN during neuroborreliosis.

Dosage: 20-30 mg zinc picolinate with copper daily.

Caution: DO NOT TAKE at the same time as you take melatonin: melatonin binds zinc (and copper). Take zinc in the morning, melatonin at night just before bed.

Melatonin

Melatonin is a natural hormone produced by the pineal gland at night; lack of light stimulates its production. Disruption of sleep cycles, aging, and some diseases with a chronic fatigue element will cause decreases, sometimes significantly, in melatonin production.

Melatonin has been found to be a potent ROS scavenger that helps reduce the synergy between QUIN and ROS in neurotoxic impacts during neuroborreliosis. Studies have found that melatonin protects brain neurons from damage by QUIN.

Melatonin can also help with the sleep disruption that often occurs in Lyme borreliosis.

Dosage: 0.6-3 mg daily. People report various effects from taking melatonin, from hyperstimulation to feeling groggy the next day with a 3 mg dose. Some people find the 0.6 mg dose effective, for others it does nothing and higher doses are necessary. It is best to begin with the smallest dose and increase it slowly after you experience your individual response to the supplement. The smallest dose I have seen for sale is 600 mcg (aka 0.6 mg), the largest appears to be 3 mg. Start with either 0.6 mg or 1 mg and see how you do for a week or so.

Caution: Take melatonin at night just before bed as it can cause grogginess. This is good as it is specific for helping Lyme-initiated sleep disruption. DO NOT TAKE at the same time you take your zinc, it will bind it. Take the zinc in the morning.

DEPRESSION

Depression is a common problem with Lyme infection. The best thing that can be done for that is a regular, weekly Swedish massage. I have used this as an adjunct to healing, both as a psychotherapist and herbalist, for over 20 years. The outcomes are remarkable (see Lymph section for more detail). It is one of the hardest things to convince people do to (too self-indulgent, they think) but the one that has the best outcome. It is far better than pharmaceutical intervention. After massage, the best thing for depression is eleutherococcus tincture.

LYME-SPECIFIC JOINT PAIN/ARTHRITIS INTERVENTION

Probably the most potent choice is *Stephania tetrandra* (See Bell's palsy listing). Teasel root has been used as well with good success in the treatment of Lyme arthritis and vitamin A has been found specific.

Teasel root (*Dipsacus sylvestris*)

Teasel root has a long history of use in Traditional Chinese Medicine (TCM). Specifically, it is used to tonify the kidney and liver, to strengthen the sinews and bones, for sore, painful knees and lower back, and weakness in the legs. It is considered to be an herb that promotes the circulation, alleviates pain, and helps recovery from chronic diseases accompanied by loss of weight. It is especially good for painful swelling or inflammation in the lower back and limbs, especially the knees. This specificity for the knees, blood circulation, and tonifying action on cartilage makes the herb very useful in Lyme disease.

Matthew Wood pioneered the use of teasel root for Lyme disease and it does help many people, sometimes considerably. The herb, as

Matthew remarks, is an excellent medicine for joint injury, especially with chronic inflammation, pain, limitations in movement, where "the person becomes arthritic, the muscles all over are stiff and sore, and they are eventually incapacitated."

A number of people with Lyme have reported that they experienced Herxheimer reactions with teasel, indicating that the herb is killing spirochetes. Treatment outcomes have, however, been mixed. Practitioners, generally on the East Coast, report less powerful impacts on spirochetes than those I have talked to in Wisconsin and Minnesota. Nearly all practitioners report that it does help with arthritic problems, pain, soreness, and movement restriction. Practitioners in the Wisconsin/Minnesota area have reported that the herb does seem to kill off spirochetes as a number of their patients have reported Herxheimer reactions with use of the herb. This outcome has not been found as much on the East Coast. The difference in outcomes between regions may be due to different strains of the spirochetes, different dosing, or different symptom pictures in patients.

Dosage: Generally used as a tincture. Matthew Wood uses tiny dosages: 1-3 drops, 1-3x daily. Other practitioners sometimes use higher dose ranges: 10-30 drops to 3x daily. The Chinese generally use 6-12 grams of the dried root daily.

Vitamin A

Vitamin A deficiency has been found to exacerbate Lyme arthritis in studies on mice. Vitamin A deficiencies have been linked to strong inflammatory responses in a number of conditions and this occurs as well in Lyme arthritis. Infected mice had a rapid vitamin A decline that correlated with the onset of arthritic symptoms. This is especially so in late-stage Lyme arthritis where the deficiency of vitamin A appears to enhance an acute arthritogenic inflammatory response initiated by IFN-gamma secretion.

Dosage: 5,000-10,000 IU daily

GENERAL ARTHRITIC SYMPTOMS AND PAIN RELIEF INTERVENTION

While many if not most of the arthritic symptoms will resolve with use of the core protocol, *Stephania spp.*, teasel root, and vitamin A the following will help as antiinflammatories and for pain relief if something extra is needed.

Devil's Claw (*Harpagophytum procumbens*)
Devil's claw is an African herb used for centuries in the treatment of arthritis. A number of clinical trials have found the herb to be as powerful as the pharmaceutical phenylbutazone in the treatment of pain and inflammation. The herb contains a constituent, harpagoside, that is specific for joint inflammation and pain.
Dosage: 1,000-2,000 mg 3x daily

> **GENERAL ARTHRITIS PROTOCOL**
>
> Curcumin/bromelain combination 400-500 mg, 3x daily).
>
> Devil's Claw: 1000-2000 mg, 3x day.
>
> Nettle: 1200 mg daily.
>
> Capsaicin cream (topical): 4x daily if needed.
>
> Arthritis tea daily

Nettle (*Urtica dioica*)
Numerous studies have found that not only does nettle possess powerful nutrients and compounds for joint and bone health it possesses specific anti-inflammatory actions as well. Historically, this entailed running the hands or affected area through living nettles, allowing the body to be "stung." Each hairlike "sting" of a nettle plant is actually a pressure-filled botanical hypodermic. Touching the sting breaks off the tip and allows the contents of the sting to be forcibly injected under the skin. The compounds in the nettle sting are similar to that in bee venom (apis) although it does not contain melittin, the most potent constituent of apis. Still, nettle compounds are strongly anti-inflammatory. Most people are not willing to sting themselves these days but the compounds can be had just as well by taking a nettle supplement.

A powerful reason for nettle's effectiveness in arthritic diseases is that it inhibits elastase. Elastase, a natural substance in the body, is used to degrade elastin, cartilage, collagen and fibronectin. This can cause serious problems in the joints, skin, and lungs if elastase activity becomes elevated, which it can do in many arthritic conditions, including Lyme disease. Nettle will inhibit the breakdown of cartilage during Lyme arthritis as well as acting as a strong anti-inflammatory.

The herb also contains high levels of boron, which the Rheumatoid Arthritis Foundation recommends (3 mg daily) for those with arthritic conditions.

Dosage: 1200 mg daily. The plant, if you have access to it fresh, can be steamed and eaten like spinach. It loses its sting on steaming or boiling. Wear gloves when harvesting. The steamed juice can be saved and used as a daily tea.

Capsaicin Cream

Capsaicin is a compound found in hot peppers (*Capsicum spp.*), that stimulates the body to release its natural pain-relieving compounds, endorphins. Several over-the-counter (OTC) creams are available that contain capsaicin (Zostrix or Capzasin-P, for example). These kinds of creams have been found to be effective in reducing arthritic pain. One study showed a reduction in rheumatoid arthritic pain by one-half and in osteoarthritic pain by one-third.

Dosage: Topical application to 4x daily if needed.

Side effects: Don't rub your eyes or touch other sensitive mucous membranes after applying these creams. Wash your hands thoroughly. If you don't, the first thing you know you will be reading a book, unconsciously rubbing an eyelid, and a few minutes later, find yourself racing for the bathroom.

Curcumin/Bromelain Combination

Curcumin is an extracted constituent of the turmeric plant that gives curry its yellow coloring. Curcumin has been found to be a highly effective anti-inflammatory in numerous studies. It has been found to be as effective as cortisone and phenylbutazone but without their side effects. Curcumin, while not addressing the exact pathways through which MMP-1, and MMP-3 inflammatory compounds are induced in Lyme arthritis is still active for MMP-1 and -3 arthritic inflammations.

Bromelain is an isolated constituent of pineapple and has been found in a number of trials to be a powerful anti-inflammatory for conditions such as bursitis and tendinitis. Studies with athletes have consistently shown reduced swelling and faster healing times with the use of bromelain. It has also been found to enhance CD57 expression which makes it useful in late-stage or chronic Lyme infections.

Dosage: These are available in many dosages both separately and together. They are, however often available in combination. The internet is a good place to look for them. Try to get 400-600 mg of curcumin daily and 250-750 mg of bromelain daily in whatever combination you come up with.

Arthritis Tea

This tea combination will help with inflammation and pain considerably and it tastes pretty nice.

Ingredients: One pound dried, cut-and-sifted (i.e., not whole or powdered) each of nettles, horsetail, dandelion leaf, peppermint leaf, celery seed, tumeric, devil's claw, and meadowsweet.

Directions: Combine all ingredients and mix well. Add one cup of the mixed herbs to one-half gallon of nearly boiling water and allow to steep covered overnight. Drink 3-4 cups daily.

Side effects: Will increase urine expression. Don't drink right before bed.

MEMORY AND COGNITIVE DYSFUNCTION

Polygonum cuspidatum (resveratrol) and *Stephania spp.* (See Bells' palsy) are the most specific for these problems as they will lessen the inflammation that is the direct cause of the problem. Interventions for Lyme neurotoxins (see listing) will offer significant help as well. And eleutherococcus can help considerably. However, if additional support is needed to deal with severe cognitive problems, the following may be of help. Zinc supplementation is indicated in any event (see neurotoxin listing).

Huperzine A (*Huperzia serratum*)

Huperzine A, a constituent of the common clubmoss *Huperzia serratum*, has a number of potent impacts on the functioning of the brain, which makes it highly useful for conditions like stroke and Alzheimer's disease. It is a neuroprotector, a neural tonic, a cholinesterase inhibitor, a butyrocholinesterase inhibitor, an anti-amnesic, is antiglaucomic, antimyasthenic, memorigenic, anti-inflammatory, a febrifuge, an antihemorrhoidal, and a capillary tonic.

> **COGNITIVE DYSFUNCTION PROTOCOL**
>
> Huperzine A, 50-100 mcg 2x day
>
> Vinpocetine, 10mg 3x day
>
> L-acetyl-carnetine, 500 mg 3x day
>
> Zinc, 40 mg day
>
> Swedish massage weekly (see "Lymph" listing)

The club moss, from which huperzine A comes, is traditionally used in Chinese medicine, where it is called either Qian Ceng Ta, meaning "thousand-layered pagoda," or Jin Bu Huan, meaning "more valuable than gold." It has been commonly used for fevers, inflammatory disorders (arthritis and rheumatism), and general vascular weakness that causes bruising, bleeding from the lungs, or hemorrhoids. A similar species, *Lycopodium clavatum*, has been used for thousands of years in Ayurvedic medicine in much the same way but also for dizziness, epilepsy, irritable bladder, and nighttime urination problems. The American Eclectic botanical physicians during the late nineteenth and early twentieth centuries also used it for urinary gravel and kidney stones. American Indians, for several thousand years, used the various lycopodiums for exactly the same things.

For millennia, in every culture in which they grow, these plants have been used for such problems as vascular insufficiency, central nervous system problems such as epilepsy and dementia, for arthritis, and for problems with nighttime urination.

In 1980, Chinese physicians isolated huperzine-A from this species, then known as *Lycopodium serratum*, and isolated huperzine-B five years later. *Huperzia serrata* contains other interesting chemicals such as the alkaloid fordine which has been found *in vivo* to possess similar actions to the huperzines—speeding up learning, reversing impaired learning, and protecting against hippocampal and cortical damage of the brain.

The two alkaloidal constituents of huperzia, huperzine-A and huperzine-B, exert potent effects on brain function; Huperzine-A being some ten times stronger than huperzine-B (which is why it is usually used). Of specific interest is the huperzines' ability to prevent the break-down of acetylcholine, prevent the destruction or deformity of neuronal networks in the hippocampus and cerebellum, and promote the dendrite outgrowth of neuronal cultures.

Huperzine-A is *brain specific*. Acetylcholine is active not only in the brain but in other parts of the body where it is also broken down much as it is in the brain. Huperzine-A works on acetylcholine *only* in the brain while at the same time protecting the breakdown of neuronal networks and promoting dendrite density and complexity. This brain-specific activity of huperzine-A causes fewer side effects than those associated with the pharmaceutical cholinesterase inhibitors that are often used for cognitive dysfunction in such diseases as Alzheimer's, and which affect acetylcholine indiscriminately throughout the body. Toxicology studies have shown that huperzine-A is nontoxic even when given at 50-100 times the human therapeutic dose. The extract also continues to be active in the brain far longer than pharmaceuticals, up to six hours at a dose (*in vivo*) of 2 mcg per kilogram (2.2 pounds) of body weight. This has been averaged to 150 mcg 2x day in clinical trials.

The research and clinical trials are impressive. One placebo-controlled, double-blind trial with 160 people suffering from Alzheimer's found huperzine A to be significantly superior to placebo, the pharmaceutical Tacrine, and another cholinesterase inhibitor, physostigmine. Huperzine A was active for three hours versus two for Tacrine and thirty minutes for physostigmine. Patients and caregivers reported significant improvement in clear-headedness, memory, and language over both placebo and other medications. In another instance, a double-blind, placebo-controlled trial was conducted with 103 people with Alzheimer's disease. Half the people were given huperzine A (100 mcg 2x daily) and half were given a placebo, for eight weeks. All participants were evaluated with the following scales: Wechsler memory, Hasegawa dementia, mini-mental state examination, activity of daily living, and treatment emergency symptom. Significant changes were seen in 58% of the people taking huperzine-A in memory, cognitive, and behavioral functions. Clinical studies have also taken place with 56 people with stroke (multi-infarct dementia) and 100 with senile memory disorders. Both studies showed significant improvement in those taking huperzine A. Another study tested huperzine-A with 34 pairs of middle school students who had complained of memory problems. One group took huperzine A (two 50 mcg capsules, 2x daily), the other a placebo for four weeks. Learning and test scores were significantly enhanced in the Huperzine group.

Dosage: Most commonly the purified extract *Huperzine A* is used, generally in 50 microgram (mcg) capsules. Typical dosage is 50-100 mcg 2x per day. (Huperzine is often found combined with other memory herbs such as ginkgo. Normally each tablet or capsule will contain a minimum of 50 mcg huperzine A.)

The whole herb itself has traditionally been used as a tincture, as a whole powder, or as a tea. No one has, to my knowledge, tried the herb by itself in the treatment of memory disorders, nor have I been able to find exactly how much huperzine A is present in sample quantities of the plant.

Caution: This herb, sometimes called Jin Bu Huan in Chinese medicine, should not be confused with the patent remedy containing tetrahydropalmatine, which is also confusingly called Jin Bu Huan.

Periwinkle (Vinpocetine) *(Vinca minor, V. major)*

The periwinkles have been used for thousands of years as herbs for stopping bleeding, for diarrhea and dysentery, nervous disorders, headaches, vertigo, and memory difficulties. A relative, the Madagascar periwinkle (*Vinca rosea*), a historical diabetic tonic, is better known today as the source of the cancer drugs vinblastine and vincristine.

Vincamine was isolated from the lesser periwinkle, *Vinca minor*, in the early 1950s and some 300 papers have been written on it since.

Vincamine has specific effects on cerebral blood flow-it increases flow, increases oxygen consumption by the brain, and enhances brain-blood-glucose utilization. Vincamine exerts a tonic effect on the cerebral arterioles and revitalizes cerebral metabolism. Double-blind trials and ECG readings have consistently shown that vincamine improves electrical activity in the brain, memory, concentration, behavior and speech disorders, irritability, vertigo, headaches, concentration, tinnitus, and blood flow in the retina of the eye.

Vincamine was withdrawn from the market by the FDA due to concerns about long term use by the elderly and children although no adverse reports existed from low dose tablet use. It has been replaced by a semi-synthetic derivative of vincamine called vinpocetine. Vinpocetine, like vincamine, enhances cerebral blood flow, acts as a neuroprotector in the CNS, is a vasodilator, and enhances memory and cognitive function. Further data is available online from numerous sources (see. e.g. http://en.wikipedia.org/wiki/Vinpocetine).

Dosage: There are a few anecdotal reports of hypersensitivity to vinpocetine in a few people. As a result a low initial dosage is recommended: 2-5 mg 3x daily with meals for a week. Then dosage can be increased. Optimum dosage is 10 mg 3x daily with a high dosage range of 40mg a day.

Side Effects: No adverse reactions have been reported in any human trial. It has been implicated in one case of agranulocytosis where granulocytes, a type of white blood cell, markedly decreases. German Commission E warns that vinpocetine, rarely, can reduce immune function and that it may cause apoptosis with long term use. None of these claims have been verified in clinical trial or study. Its safety in pregnancy has not been determined.

L-acetylcarnitine (LAC)

L-acetylcarnitine (LAC) is naturally present in the brain and researchers have found that it mimics the actions of acetylcholine. To some extent, LAC acts like an acetylcholine supplement. In at least six placebo-controlled trials with Alzheimer's patients, LAC was found to consistently improve function in all the areas studied, including memory, cognition, and behavior. Other studies with age-related mental impairment found the same kinds of improvement. Dosage range in most of the studies was 1,500 to 2,000 mg per day.

Dosage: 500 mg, 3x day.

Zinc

A number of studies have found that zinc levels are chronically low in aging populations. Zinc levels in Alzheimer's patients are often extremely low. There has been some preliminary evidence that the neurofibrillary tangles in the brains of Alzheimer's patients are exacerbated by zinc deficiencies. One controlled study with ten Alzheimer's patients found that eight improved significantly with 27 mg of zinc supplementation, one 79-year-old man miraculously so.

Dosage: 40 mg day.

ANGINA AND HEART PROBLEMS

Many of the core protocol herbs will help this directly. If they are insufficient, vincamine will help as well. The following can also be used.

PROTOCOL FOR ANGINA AND HEART PROBLEMS

Astragalus, 1,000 to 4,000 mg, 3-4x daily (See core protocol)

Hawthorn, 120-900 mg 3x daily.

Khella, 250-300 mg daily

L-Carnitine-500 mg 3x day

Hawthorn (*Crataegus oxyacantha*)

The berries of the hawthorn bush (and sometimes the leaves and flowers) have been used as a heart tonic for at least 2,000 years in western medicine and for a bit less than 700 in China. They are specific for nearly every manifestation of heart disease: atherosclerosis, cardiac arrhythmia, congestive heart failure, hypertension, and peripheral vascular disease.

In vivo studies have found that the herb lowers blood pressure, increases blood vessel dilation throughout the body, lowers cholesterol levels in the blood, and is powerfully antiarrhythmic, slowing and normalizing heart beat.

Both *in vivo* and *in vitro* studies have shown that hawthorn increases both the amplitude of heart contractions and its stroke volume. Studies also show that if blood pressure is too low, hawthorn raises it, if it is too high, hawthorn lowers it. It is in fact a normalizer of blood pressure and a regulator of blood flow within the body.

While substances like adrenaline or digoxin increase the heart's rate and beat strength in order to increase blood flow in the body, hawthorn lowers heart rate and still accomplishes the same thing. With hawthorn, muscular contractions of the heart are slower, longer, and more powerful. This particular type of beating pattern is associated with higher ANF levels, more relaxed states, and lower cortisol levels—basically an anabolic pattern. Adrenaline, on the other hand, is a catabolic heart stimulant. Hawthorn is virtually the only anabolic heart medicine known.

Dozens of clinical trials have been conducted with hawthorn extracts on thousands of people with heart disease. All have confirmed the herb's remarkable effectiveness. In one study, 300 mg of the dried leaf was taken daily in a placebo-controlled, double-blind trial of 46 men with angina. After four weeks angina had been reduced in all patients by 86%. Another study with 78 people with congestive heart failure were given 600 mg daily of hawthorn for eight weeks. Exercise tolerance significantly increased; heart rate and blood pressure both significantly decreased. Another study showed that 87% of participants in a hawthorn trial experienced lower cholesterol levels, 80% had lower triglycerides. All experienced lower blood pressure and more dilation in coronary vessels. In another trial, 1,011 people were given a standardized extract, 900 mg, for 24 weeks. A significant improvement was seen in exercise tolerance, fatigue levels, palpitation, and dyspnea. Ankle edema and nocturia were reduced by 83%. A more stable heart rate and reductions in blood pressure were common. A significant reduction in the number of people with ST depression, arrhythmia, and ventricular extrasystole was seen.

Part of the reason that hawthorn reduces cholesterol is that it literally repairs the cellular structure of blood vessel walls. Hawthorn contains *procyanidins*, a flavonoid complex similar to those found in bilberry (anthocyanosides) and pine bark and grape seed (proanthocyanidins—aka PCOs).

Procyanidins protect collagen fibers from damage, increase their elasticity, and reinforce the cross-linking of collagen fibers to make them stronger and hence make the blood vessels less prone to cracking. Procyanidins increase intracellular vitamin C levels (which is necessary for collagen synthesis), stimulate circulation to peripheral blood vessels, are potent antioxidants, and are strongly anti-inflammatory. They also lower cell-membrane permeability and help protect cellular integrity. *All these functions are exceptionally supportive in Lyme disease. They will considerably help to reduce symptoms.*

Hawthorn also has a direct effect on the diameter of blood vessels and arteries, causing them to dilate. This increases the oxygen being received by the heart. Hawthorn also changes the rhythm and pattern of the heart beat. The heart beats slower, the beats last longer, and the power is increased. The longer the herb is used the more healing that occurs in vessel walls and the more toned the muscle of the heart becomes.

Dosage: 120-900 mg of the herb daily or one fourth to one half teaspoon 3x daily of the tincture.

The dosage range in most clinical studies has been from 120-900 mg daily. Most of these have used non-standardized (i.e. raw herb) extracts, either in capsules or as an alcoholic tincture. Some practitioners are suggesting that the extracts be standardized for 1.8% vitexin-4'-rhamnoside or 10% procyanidin content. Not everyone agrees. The herb is effective in both forms and a number of people feel that the herb is most efficacious in whole form without the seemingly inevitable human tinkering.

Khella (*Amni visnaga*)

Khella has been used in Egypt for some four to six thousand years for the treatment of heart disease and angina, one of the few herbs that has come out of ancient Egyptian tradition. Khella works fairly rapidly to dilate the coronary arteries, increasing blood supply to the heart. Scores of clinical trials have explored the herb and one of its constituents *khellin*. It was endorsed by the *New England Journal of Medicine* in 1951 as a safe and effective treatment for angina pectoris. Normally, the herb is found standardized for its khellin content, 12%.

Dosage: 250-300 mg daily.

Contraindications and side effects: Khellin can cause skin sensitivity to light and caution should be exercised by fair-skinned people, especially if you spend any time in the sun. Because this is sometimes a problem from the antibiotics used in treating Lyme and Lyme infection, as well, caution should be exercised in the use of this herb. In rare instances, the herb may cause mild liver inflammation or jaundice. These conditions clear when the herb is discontinued.

L-Carnitine

In a significant number of trials, carnitine has been found to relieve angina, increase exercise times, improve energy levels, reduce heart disease, and protect the heart from damage. As oxygen levels to the heart fall because of occlusion, carnitine levels also fall. Reduced carnitine leads to a number of problems as it is essential in heart muscle for healthy functioning.

Dosage: 500 mg 3x day

EYE PROBLEMS

Lyme spirochetes invade the aqueous humor of the eye almost immediately. This is one of the reasons that so many people with Lyme report "floaters" in their visual field. That the spirochetes enter this part of the body makes treatment more difficult as antibiotics are slow to work in this area. The core protocol should help eye problems considerably. However, many of the symptoms of Lyme infection—fuzzy vision, pressure in the eye, and so on—can also be helped by the herbs and supplements listed here. In some respects, Lyme infection of the humor of the eye creates a kind of mild glaucoma. The breakdown of collagen and the inflammation from the bacterial infection are similar to some of the processes that occur in that condition.

Glaucoma is an increase in the amount of the internal fluid of the

PROTOCOL FOR EYE PROBLEMS

Stephania root, one-half teaspoon
of the tincture 3x daily, eye wash
with decoction.

Vinpocetine, 10 mg 3x daily

Vitamin C, 1,000 mg 3x daily
(effervescent salts)

Zinc, 40 mg daily

eye that creates a pressure inside the eyeball. Fuzzy vision is one of the symptoms. Collagen deterioration is strongly involved. In essence, the collagen in the eye breaks down and is not processed properly so it builds up in the fluid of the eye. This blocks the drainage of intraocular fluid out of the eye creating increased interior pressure. As pressure increases, the optic nerve can be damaged. This causes blurred vision, loss of peripheral vision, halo effects around lights, blind spots, eye pain, and redness (all more acute conditions than those that generally occur in Lyme disease).

Probably the best herb for eye problems associated with Lyme disease is stephania root (See Bell's palsy). Vinpocetine can be exceptionally helpful as well. Vitamin C will help support the eye's collagen structures and zinc is also specific.

MUSCLE TWITCHES
TINGLING/CRAWLING SENSATION IN SKIN

These are sometimes reported by people with Lyme disease. The core protocol can help considerably but if the problems persist, the following have been found to be helpful. Please note that vitamin B-12 and magnesium deficiency are both common in chronic Lyme infections. Muscle twitches and a tingling or crawling sensation in the skin are two of the primary symptoms of these kinds of deficiencies. Both are important to address. The magnesium deficiency contributes as well to heart problems; common aspects are hyperreflexia, muscle twitches, myocardial irritability, poor stamina, and muscle spasms and seizures, especially in the legs. In general, a good B-complex formula is essential in Lyme infections as well.

Warning: Magnesium should be used with caution and under a health care provider's supervision if high-grade atrioventricular block is a possibility.

> **PROTOCOL FOR MUSCLE TWITCHES**
>
> Vitamin B-12, 1,000 mcg daily (lower to 500 mcg as symptoms resolve)
>
> Vitamin B-6, 100 mg 2x daily (lower to 50 mg as symptoms resolve)
>
> Folic acid, 400 mcg daily
>
> Magnesium, 200-400 mg to 3x daily

SWOLLEN LYMPH NODES OR SLUGGISH LYMPH SYSTEM:

The immune system will work hard to deal with the Lyme infection but as dead bacteria accumulate they—and used-up cells from the immune response—will be taken to the lymph system for disposal. As a result, the lymph system tends to clog up during acute infections. This is, in part, why the lymph nodes swell. It is like a highway clogged by too many cars in rush hour. The more efficiently the lymph system cleans out the garbage the more potent your immune response will be. In addition, certain parts of the lymph system actually potentiate immune responses. The best general herb for lymph support is red root (*Ceanothus spp.*). In acute conditions, sometimes the lymph system is so sluggish it needs considerable pushing. At such times, poke root (*Phytolacca decandra*) is indicated, three to five drops 3x day. This is a much stronger herb than red root and should be used with caution. If you are not knowledgeable about poke, using it under a practitioner's direction is best. Massage is also exceptionally good for a sluggish lymph system.

> **SLUGGISH OR SWOLLEN LYMPH SYSTEM**
>
> Red root tincture, full dropper 3x daily
>
> Swedish massage weekly

Red Root (*Ceanothus americanus* or equivalent)

First and foremost red root is a lymph-system stimulant and tonic. It is strongly anti-inflammatory for both the liver and spleen. It is also an astringent, a mucous membrane tonic, alterative, antiseptic, expectorant, antispasmodic, and an exceptionally strong blood coagulant.

Red root is an important herb in that it helps facilitate clearing of dead cellular tissue from the lymph system. When the immune system is responding to acute conditions or the onset of disease, as white blood cells kill disease pathogens they are taken to the lymph system for disposal. When the lymph system can clear out dead cellular material rapidly, the healing process is increased, sometimes dramatically. The herb shows especially strong action whenever any portion of the lymph system is swollen, infected, or inflamed. This includes lymph nodes, tonsils, spleen, appendix, and liver. There is some evidence that red root's activity in the lymph nodes also enhances the lymph nodes' production of lymphocytes, specifically the formation of T cells. Clinicians working with AIDS patients, who have historically low levels of T cells, have noted increases after the use of red root. Nineteenth-century western botanic medicine used the herb to reduce inflammations in the liver and spleen.

A number of human trials have occurred using the herb as a tincture extract (usually 10-15 ml per person). The trials focused on heavy bleeding, including excess menstruation, and red root was found to be a powerful coagulant and hemostatic in all studies. A marked reduction of clotting time was noted. *In vivo* studies have shown marked hemostatic activity and hypotensive action. *In vitro* studies have also shown a strong reverse transcriptase inhibition and a broad antifungal activity.

Dosage in Lyme Disease: Tincture: dry root, 1:5 50% alcohol, 30-90 drops to 4x day.

Side Effects and Contraindications: No side effects have been noted. However, red root is contraindicated in people using blood coagulants or anticoagulants and in pregnancy.

Swedish Massage

A Swedish massage, like most massages usually lasts from one to one-and-a-half hours. During that time, a good practitioner can relieve a majority of the tension and stress that people commonly hold in their bodies. Each person holds tension in different places—wrists, forearms, shoulders, neck, back, etc. As your massage therapist gets to know you, they become more and more efficient in helping reduce body-held tension. This produces a number of benefits including reduced anxiety, deeper respiration, less tendency to become depressed, enhanced immune function, and increased mental alertness.

The lymph system of the body, a parallel circulatory system to the blood, does not have a muscular pump to keep things moving. Instead, the lymph system is "worked" by the movement of the muscles. The lymph system moves white blood cells and cellular debris, especially the debris that occurs during disease, through and out of the body. One of the reasons that the lymph nodes swell during disease is that they are filled with old white blood cells and dead bacteria. The more efficiently the lymph system moves dead bacteria and old white blood cells, the more quickly people get well. Some form of movement of the muscles of the body is needed for the lymph system to remain healthy. In addition to stimulating the health of the lymph system, massage has been shown to produce direct increases in white blood cell and other immuno-active cells of the immune system. Other physiological alterations include a 10%-15% increase in oxygen capacity of the blood after a massage, increased excretion of nitrogen, phosphorus, and salt in the urine, and improved skin health.

In addition to its impacts on the lymph system, there are a number of major health benefits to massage. These include regular intimate human contact, enhanced immune function, lowered blood pressure, reduced anxiety, deeper respiration, less depression, improved alertness, reduced heart rate, reduced tension levels, increased blood circulation, enhanced joint flexibility and range of motion, lower pain levels in chronic disease

MUSCLE WEAKNESS AND LACK OF STRENGTH

The following tincture is best taken after the worst of the Lyme conditions have started to resolve, when there is lingering weakness. It will help restore muscle tone and strength after long-term chronic illness and fatigue.

Combine equal parts of the tinctures of pine pollen, *Aralia naudicaulis*, and American ginseng. Take a full dropper of the tincture 3x daily for six months. (Available from Woodland Essence: www.woodlandessence.com or 315-845-1515.)

TO KILL CANDIDA:

Capryl (SolarRay brand) 2163 mg caprylic acid, 2 caps 3x daily. Undecenoic acid, Thorne Research Formula SF722, 50 mg, 2 gel caps 3x daily. (Both caprylic and undecenoic acids are strongly inhibitive to candida organisms.)

TO ENHANCE BOWEL/SYSTEM NORMALIZATION:

Thymic Formula (Preventative Therapeutics) 2 tablets, 3x daily.

Molybdenum picolinate, 1,000 mcg, 1 capsule daily.

TO RESTORE BOWEL FLORA:

PB8 (probiotic acidophilus capsules), 2 capsules daily.

Saccharomyces boulardii, one capsule 3x daily

CANDIDA OVERGROWTH

Many people with Lyme, after having taken long courses of antibiotics, have abnormal bowel flora, often candida overgrowth. These supplements will kill most of the candida and support the normalization of bowel flora.

MAINTAINING INTESTINAL HEALTH ON ANTIBIOTICS

This will keep bowel function healthy when on long term antibiotics and will reduce diarrhea and other complications considerably while normalizing function.

PB8 (probiotic acidophilus capsules), 2 capsules daily.

CHRONIC FATIGUE

Chronic fatigue is a serious problem with many long-term illnesses and Lyme disease is no exception. Numerous studies have found severe, persistent chronic fatigue as a common element in Lyme infections, especially in people who live or have lived in endemic areas. (See for example, Coyle et al. "Borrelia burgdorferi reactivity in patients with severe chronic fatigue who are from a region in which Lyme disease is endemic." *Clin Infect Dis* 1994 Jan;18(suppl):S24-7.) Many of those who have been infected experience their disease, in spite of multiple antibiotic regimens, as a chronic condition much like malaria. They are fine for long periods with regular relapses marked by severe fatigue. These bouts of fatigue normally last several days and are incapacitating. While pharmaceuticals are inefficient at treating chronic fatigue, plant medicines are exceptionally good. The use of the herbs in the core protocol should help immensely, especially the andrographis and astragalus. However, if after having used them for awhile, chronic fatigue is still a problem, or if you have acute onset with severe fatigue, or if you have been previously treated and have no other symptoms except periodic bouts of chronic fatigue, eleutherococcus (Siberian ginseng) is specifically indicated. Weekly massage is also exceptionally good for this condition and in some twenty years of practice I have seen it help consistently in chronic fatigue conditions; it is a primary recommendation for this problem. It will permanently reverse the problem over time—unless you suffer an extended period of unremittant stress. This will tend to stimulate relapses until the stressors are relieved.

For the most detail on the use of eleuthero see "Acute Onset."

TREATMENT OF CHRONIC FATIGUE IN LYME DISEASE

Core protocol for Lyme disease

Eleuthero tincture, 2-3
  teaspoons daily for 60 days

Swedish massage weekly

However, if you suffer periodic bouts of chronic fatigue without other symptoms, keep a bottle of Herb Pharm eleuthero tincture on hand. (No other brands, if they are not at least a 1:1 formulation, will do.) If you then wake up with the all-too-familiar malaise and severe fatigue, begin taking two teaspoons of the tincture in water daily— one teaspoon in the morning when you rise and another at lunch. You can take another before dinner if you wish, but it can cause sleeplessness. You can take up to an ounce of the tincture daily. This will normally reverse this kind of periodic chronic fatigue within 24-48 hours. (See "Acute Onset" for dosage and contraindication information.)

HEADACHES

Herbs already discussed will help considerably with the headaches that come with Lyme infection or and its coinfectious agents. For reducing the inflammation in the meninges that cause them: *Polygonum cuspidatum* and *Stephania*. For helping with the headaches themselves through other mechanisms: *Andrographis* and Vinpocetine.

CHAPTER FIVE

Treatment of
Lyme Coinfections

☙

Ticks that carry Lyme disease often carry other infectious agents as well. The most common are babesia, ehrlichia, and bartonella.

The number of ticks coninfected with organisms other than Lyme borrelia tends to run anywhere from 2% to 26% in heavily infected areas. Coinfection rates in people have been found to be between 39% and 60% in some Lyme-endemic areas. Babesia coinfections tend to occur most often (at least at this point in time). About 80% of people who are coinfected at the time of tick bite have been found to have babesia in addition to Lyme. Ehrlichia occurs in about 3%-15% of those with coinfections, and bartonella in less than 5%. Very rarely there can be coinfections by other organisms such as tick borne encephalitis (TBE), Chlamydia trachomatis, and Rocky Mountain Spotted Fever. The incidence of TBE coinfection, for example, in Slovenia is about one person every five years. Rocky Mountain Spotted fever (RMSF) is in the same family as ehrlichia organisms, and infection with ehrlichia is sometimes referred to as spotless Rocky Mountain fever.

The tick coinfection rates for these organisms are, however, in flux, and there are indications these rates of coinfection are highly variable from year to year and location to location. A recent examination of ticks in New Jersey found that coinfection of tested ticks by both borrelia and bartonella organisms were about the same (34% of ticks tested), while ehrlicha and babesia organisms were present in many fewer ticks (2% and 8% respectively).

All three of these coinfectious agents are considered to be emerging infections. All three have been recognized as unique epidemiological agents only since 1990; research on them is very recent and not very deep. A great deal is unknown. Compounding their relative newness, they have been difficult to grow in laboratory settings making them much harder to study. Finding effective treatment regimens has, as a result, also been more difficult. Antibiotics do work in many instances, but even less is known about these infections' relapse rates, long-term impacts, and subtleties of antibiotic application in treating them than is known about Lyme borreliosis. What is clear, however, is that the severity of the diseases caused by each of these organisms increases if there is a coinfection with Lyme spirochetes. The impacts of the Lyme spirochetes and the severity of Lyme symptoms increases as well. The organisms are highly synergistic with each other.

What we are seeing, in effect, are the beginnings of epidemic. endemic infections in human populations of synergistic coinfectious agents.

These three coinfectious agents add an additional layer of complexity to an already complex disease process. The symptom picture of Lyme is altered in unique ways when any of these coinfections are present. Primarily symptoms are much worse and resolution takes much longer.

In any treatment of Lyme borreliosis, it is important to realize that coinfection may exist. Relapse rates are higher if coinfections are present and antibiotics are less effective. Symptom resolution is more difficult as well. Practitioners on the front lines have found that, in the case of babesia for example, the babesia must be treated first in order to bring the Lyme infection under control more successfully.

The following treatment protocols are specific for babesia, ehrlichia, and bartonella, the three primary coinfectious agents of Lyme disease.

BABESIA

Babesia is a protozoal parasite, much like malaria, except that instead of mosquitos it is transmitted by ticks. Like malarial parasites, babesia protozoa infect red blood cells and eventually destroy them. The symptoms of the disease are, as a result, very similar to malaria.

The same ecosystem species that support populations of Lyme spirochetes and their associated ticks—white-footed mice and deer—also maintain and transmit babesia organisms in the wild. Coinfection with Lyme and babesia will be with us a long time.

There are 13 different forms of babesia. Only three regularly infect people (though a few others sometimes find their way into our systems). They are: *Babesia microti* in the central and eastern United States, *WA-1* in the western United States, and *Babesia divergens* in Europe.

Testing is problematical. Tests only look for these three babesia species. If you are infected with another type, the test will come up negative. Compounding the problem, like Lyme, the tests are not completely accurate. Blood smears are only reliable for the first two weeks of infection; the tests are not sensitive enough for later or mild infections. Thus there are a lot of false negatives.

Babesiosis is now considered an emerging disease in the United States and is recognized to be endemic in a number of areas. It has gained recognition primarily because of its tendency to occur as a coinfection in Lyme disease. The antibiotics normally used for Lyme spirochetes are generally not effective against babesia organisms.

The symptoms of babesia infection generally include a vague sense of imbalance, headache, fatigue, anorexia, muscle and joint pain, feelings of chest compression, shortness of breath, chills/fever, nausea, malaise, and drenching sweats. If the lungs become involved, cough is sometimes present.

Coinfection with Lyme spirochetes, however, causes the symptoms and impacts of both diseases to be more acute and severe. Symptoms can then include severe headaches, hemolytic anemia, central-nervous-system involvement, high fevers, and shaking chills.

Lyme and babesia organisms have been found to act in a synergistic manner. Spirochete DNA is more evident and remains in circulation longer when babesia infection is also present. Impacts on joints, heart, and nerves are worse and arthritic symptoms are much more severe. Transverse myelitis (inflammation of the spinal cord with arm and leg impairment) has been reported in some cases of coinfection. Illness at onset is more acute and convalescence takes longer while the array of symptoms is much broader.

With babesia infection, capillary blockage and microvascular stasis can occur as a result of red blood-cell fragments clogging the system. The liver, kidneys, and spleen may become inflamed trying to deal with the red blood-cell fragments in the vascular system. The spleen seems especially hard hit as it is primarily responsible for removing the fragments. Because of this, herbs for spleen and liver support can help considerably in the treatment of babesiosis.

The primary herb useful in the treatment of babesia is *Artemisia annua*. The use of one of the herb's constituents, artemisinin, has shown much better outcomes than the herb itself in treating babesia infections (although this may be because of too-low dosing with the whole herb).

The use of artemisinin for babesia was pioneered by Qing Cai Zhang in New York City as an adjunct in his treatment of Lyme disease. Subsequent *in vitro* studies (and substantial practitioner success) have strongly supported the herb's effectiveness. Dr. Zhang's form of artemisia is called arteannuin, which is an older term for artemisinin. Technically, artemisinin is arteannuin A. There is also an arteannuin B in the whole herb along with a considerable number of other compounds. The whole herb will work, it just takes more effort to make it work. It must be prepared as teas (generally) and the dosage must match that used in the clinical studies for the treatment of malaria (discussed in the dosage section below).

TREATMENT OF BABESIA COINFECTION

Artemisinin capsules: 100 mg 3x daily for 30-40 days

Red root (Ceanothus spp) tincture: one-half to one and one-half teaspoons (30-90 drops) to 4x day

For shaking chills/ sweats/fevers: boneset tea, 2-4 cups daily.

Treating babesia coinfection first will generally promote better outcomes in the treatment of Lyme disease.

ARTEMISININ (*Artemisia annua*)

Common names: Sweet annie, Sweet wormwood (English), Qing-hao (Chinese).

Family: *Asteraceae*

Habitat: The plant is native to China, western Asia, and southeast Europe. An emerging invasive plant species, it is naturalized in the United States, especially in Lyme endemic areas. Loves waste areas—roadsides, fallow fields, neglected gardens, especially in eastern North America. The plant is stronger and more aromatic when grown in poor, dry soil.

Collection: The plants grow 4-6 feet tall (1.2-1.8m) with a typical, attractive weedy look. They bloom in late summer. The aerial parts should be harvested just before flowering. The top third of the plant is strongest in artemisinin content.

Cultivation: Easily from seed. Sow outdoors in fall or from seed indoors before last frost. Self sows and will never go away once established.

Part used: Aerial parts, primarily the upper third of the plant, which is highest in artemisinin content.

Medicinal actions of artemisinin: Antimalarial, antiparasitical, antitumor, antiviral, calcium antagonist, immunomodulator, plasmodicide, schizonticide, antispirochetal (*in vitro*). Broadly active against dermatophytes—fungi that cause infections in hair, skin, and nails. The whole herb has a much broader range of actions than artemisinin, the isolated constituent.

Functions in Lyme disease: Primarily for the treatment of babesia coinfections. Possesses mild antiendotoxin effects that can help in reducing Herxheimer reactions. Some clinical evidence exists for the plant possibly being effective against borrelia organisms.

About *Artemisia annua* and artemisinin: Although other artemisias have been used to treat malaria, the most potent plant for this is *Artemisia annua*. It is the only plant in the family that has been found to contain artemisinin, the most active antimalarial constituent.

The plant has been used in Chinese medicine for over 2000 years but its current status as an antimalarial emerged from its use by the North Vietnamese during the Vietnam war. Malarial infections were exceptionally high among the North Vietnamese troops. Appeals to the Chinese leader, Mao Tse-tung, for help resulted in the discovery of *Artemisia annua* for use as an antimalarial.

Chinese researchers had discovered that in one region of China the people had few or no incidences of malaria. Looking closer they discovered that the local people took the herb at the first sign of symptoms. In 1972, Chinese researchers isolated artemisinin.

Ayurveda: This plant is unknown in India, although a number of other artemisias are used.

Traditional Chinese medicine: The herb is used for clearing fevers from the blood especially in conditions with headache, dizziness, low fever, and a stifling sensation in the chest. For febrile diseases with fever, for malaria.

Western botanic practice: Unknown, although many other artemisias have long been used, some for malarial conditions.

Scientific: A slightly modified form of artemisinin, artesunate, has been found effective for babesia organisms *in vitro*. Relatively low concentrations of the compound are effective; complete inhibition of *Babesia equi* and *B. caballi* occurred at 0.2 and 1.0 mcg/ml respectively.

To make artesunate, artemisinin is modified slightly in order to get patent protection; artemisinin is just as effective. Practitioners and those who have used artemisinin in the treatment of babesia have reported that it is a potent choice for treatment, and more reliable than pharmaceuticals.

Artemisinin is also effective against *Neospora caninum*, another type of protozoa that effects both endothelial cells and macrophages. Central nervous system involvement and carditis are common. It is effective against a number of other organisms such as *Eimeria tenella*, *Leishmania major* (which infects macrophages), *Toxoplasma gondii*,

Schistosoma mansoni (liver flukes), and *Clonorchia sinensis* (liver flukes)—all parasitical organisms. It is antispirochetal against leptospira organisms, killing them in *in vitro* tests. Artemisinin does appear to possess broad antiparasitical actions; its most potent impacts so far have been seen in the treatment of malaria.

There have been a significant number of clinical studies and trials on the use of both the whole herb and the isolated constituent, artemisinin, in the treatment of malaria. All have shown that both are significantly effective in the treatment of the disease. Artemisinin has become the choice for malarial treatment worldwide because it is also effective against resistant strains of the organism. Ninety-eight percent of malarial parasites are generally killed within 24 hours with use of the herb or its constituent. If low, short term doses are used, however, relapse rates can be as high as 39%. Higher dose ranges lower the relapse rate considerably. Clinical trials with as many as 2000 people (with both low and high dosages) have found 100% clearance rates for all participants.

The herb is exceptionally potent in that it spreads quickly throughout the body and it easily crosses the blood/brain barrier. Because it infuses the blood, it is carried throughout the body to every cell, all of which need blood to live. Thus, artemisinin and the whole-herb constituents produce effects extensively throughout the body.

Artemisinin possesses a broad antiparasitic action and may indeed be more potent in the treatment of Lyme disease than is currently recognized. Given its range of action and pervasive spread in the body, there is reason to suspect that, when it is comprehensively tested, it will be found effective against borrelia organisms and possibly bartonella and ehrlichia coinfectious agents as well.

Artemisinin, like many of the herbs and constituents effective in the treatment of Lyme disease, is also stimulating interest as an antitumor and anticancer compound. It has shown effectiveness as an anticancer agent both *in vitro* and *in vivo*. *In vitro* studies have found artemisinin effective against human leukemia cells, breast cancer, and colon cancer. Treatment of both bone cancer and cancer of the lymph nodes in dogs was effective with 10-15 days of treatment. The use of artemisinin in people with cancer has shown effectiveness as well. Vietnamese doctors have found it successful in curing 50%-60% of several different types of cancer patients.

Artemisinin has also shown antiendotoxin effects *in vitro*. It is broadly antifungal and antiviral.

Dosage in Lyme disease: 300-500 mg daily for 30-40 days.

Artemisinin is generally sold in 100 mg capsules. The dosage level in Lyme disease has tended to be a bit lower than for malaria and for much longer: one 100 mg capsule 3x daily for 30-40 days.

The effective dosage for malaria is 500-1000 mg on the first day and 500 mg daily thereafter for four more days. This will completely clear the malarial parasite from the blood. However, at 400 mg day for five days the recurrence rate is 39%. Dosage at 800 mg drops the recurrence rate to nearer 3% which is perhaps why dosage in China is higher—800 mg to 1600 mg per day for three days, repeated again in two weeks.

Artemisinin in whole-herb preparations: The amount of artemisinin in the aerial parts of the plant varies during the time of year and from location to location. In general, one quart (liter) of a water infusion of nine grams of *Artemisia annua* tops (one third of an ounce) harvested prior to flowering will contain about 95 mg of artemisinin. This is one fifth the daily dose needed to treat malaria or one-third of that used to treat babesia. The whole herb can reliably be used for malaria IF the dosage is increased to the 500 mg range. This would apply to babesia treatment as well. Remember, the reason this herb was discovered was that in the region of China where it is used, there were no incidences of malaria. The secret is in the dose, as with all medications.

Side effects: Artemisinin in high doses can cause gastrointesintal upset—loss of appetite, nausea, cramping, diarrhea, vomiting. Very high doses (5000 mg day of artemisinin for three days) have caused liver inflammation. It resolves upon discontinuing the herb.

Contraindications: Should be used with caution in pregnancy, especially in the first trimester.

RED ROOT (*Ceanothus americanus* or equivalent)

Family: *Rhamnaceae*

Part used: The root or inner bark of the root. The various species of red root can be used interchangeably.

Collection and habitat: Species seemingly grow everywhere and are widely divergent in appearance. The root should be harvested in the fall or early spring, whenever the root has been subjected to a good frost. The inner bark of the root is a bright red and this color extends through the white woody root as a pink tinge after a freeze. The root is extremely tough when it dries. It should be cut into small one or two inch pieces with plant snips while still fresh or you will regret it.

Actions: First and foremost a lymph system stimulant and tonic. Red root is anti-inflammatory for both the liver and spleen. It is also an astringent, a mucous membrane tonic, alterative, antiseptic, expectorant, antispasmodic, and an exceptionally strong blood coagulant.

Functions in babesia treatment: Reducing inflammation in the spleen and the liver, stimulating lymph system clearance and drainage, enhancing immune response to infection.

About red root: Red root is an important herb in that it helps facilitate clearing of dead cellular tissue from the lymph system. When the immune system is responding to acute conditions or the onset of disease as white blood cells kill disease pathogens, they are taken to the lymph system for disposal. When the lymph system can clear out dead cellular material rapidly, the healing process is increased, sometimes dramatically. The herb shows especially strong action whenever any portion of the lymph system is swollen, infected, or inflamed. This includes lymph nodes, tonsils (entire back of throat), spleen, appendix, and liver. There is some evidence that red root's activity in the lymph nodes also enhances the lymph nodes' production of lymphocytes, specifically the formation of T cells. Clinicians working with AIDS patients, who have historically low levels of T cells, have noted increases after the use of red root. It is especially effective in reducing inflammations in the spleen and liver from such things as excessive bacterial garbage, white blood-cell detritus in the lymph, and red blood cell fragments in the blood in diseases like babesiosis.

A number of human trials have occurred using the herb as a tincture extract (usually 10-15 ml per person). The trials focused on heavy bleeding, including excess menstruation and red root was found to be a powerful coagulant and hemostatic in all studies. A marked reduction of clotting time was noted. *In vivo* studies have shown marked hemostatic activity and hypotensive action. *In vitro* studies have also found a strong reverse transcriptase inhibition and a broad antifungal activity.

Dosage on babesia coinfection: Tincture: dry root, 1:5 50% alcohol, 30-90 drops to 4x day.

Side effects and contraindications: No side effects have been noted. However, it is contraindicated in people using blood coagulants or anticoagulants and in pregnancy.

BONESET (*Eupatorium perfoliatum*)

Family: *Compositae*

Part used: Above-ground plant.

Collection: If collected at flowering and allowed to dry, the plant will usually go to seed. It should only be collected in flower (August or September) if being tinctured fresh. Otherwise, it should be picked just prior to flowering, hung upside down in a shaded place, and allowed to thoroughly air-dry.

Constituents: The immunostimulants methylglucuronoxylan, astragalin, eufoliatin, euroliatorin, eupatorin, euperfolin, and euperfolitin, and a bunch of other stuff.

Actions: Immunostimulant (increases phagocytosis to 4x that of echinacea), diaphoretic, febrifuge, mucous membrane tonic, smooth muscle relaxant, antiinflammatory, cytotoxic, mild emetic, peripheral circulatory stimulant, gastric bitter, mild antibacterial.

Functions in babesia and bartonella coninfections: Boneset is exceptionally useful in both babesia and bartonella coinfections. It stimulates the immune system, normalizes the CD4/CD8 ratio, actively protects bone marrow macrophages, and stimulates their production. The herb reduces the incidence and severity of periodic fevers, pains, and disease symptoms.

About boneset: The plant, indigenous to North America, has been used by Native peoples for millennia, specifically for intermittent fevers and chills, with pain in the bones, weakness and debility.

Clinical trials have shown that boneset stimulates phagocytosis better than echinacea, is analgesic (at least as effective as aspirin), and reduces cold and flu symptoms. In mice it has shown strong immunostimulant activity and cytotoxic action against cancer cells.

Despite boneset's long use and potent reputation little research has occurred with the plant. In clinical practice, however, it is one of the most potent herbs for enhancing immune function especially in periodic diseases like bartonellosis. It will reliably counter bacterial or viral immune-suppression in diseases that present as periodics.

Dosage during coinfections: One cup of the mildly hot tea, 2-4x daily for as long as necessary: usually two to six weeks. I find the tea a more potent form of the herb for these kinds of conditions. I am not sure that the tincture form provides the kind of immunostimulation that the tea is so well-known for.

Preparation and dosages: May be taken as tea or tincture.

As tea:

Cold: One ounce of herb in quart boiling water, let steep overnight, strain and drink throughout day. The cold infusion is better for the mucous membrane system and as a liver tonic.

Hot: One teaspoon herb in eight ounces hot water, steep 15 minutes. Take four to six ounces of the hot tea to 4x per day. Boneset is only diaphoretic when hot, and should be consumed hot for active infections or for recurring chills and fevers.

Tincture: Fresh herb in flower 1:2 95% alcohol, 20-40 drops to 3x day in hot water. Dry herb: 1:5 60% alcohol, 30-50 drops in hot water to 3x day. In acute viral or bacterial upper respiratory infections: 10 drops of tincture in hot water every half-hour to 6x day. In chronic conditions where the acute stage has passed but there is continued chronic fatigue and relapse: 10 drops of tincture in hot water 4x day.

Side effects and contraindications: The hot infusion in quantity can cause vomiting, in moderate doses mild nausea sometimes occurs. The cooler the tea the less nausea. Otherwise, no side effects or contraindications.

EHRLICHIA

Ehrlichia organisms are small, gram-negative bacteria that usually invade leukocytes—white blood cells. The diseases they cause are usually named for the type of white blood cell they invade. Generally there are two: human granulocytic ehrlichiosis (HGE) and human monocytic ehrlichiosis (HME). These two diseases are caused by different but closely related organisms—*Anaplasma phagocytophila* (formerly known as *Ehrlichia phagocytophila*) in the case of HGE and *Ehrlichia chaffeensis* in HME. Two others sometimes infect people: *Ehrlichia ewingii*, which formerly only infected dogs, is now found in immunocompromised people such as those with AIDS, and *Ehrlichia sennetsu*, which is generally restricted to Japan and Malaysia.

E. *chaffeenis* infects mononuclear leukocytes (monocytes and macrophages) and A. *phagocytophila* generally infects neutrophils.

Ehrlichiosis, along with Lyme and babesiosis, is considered an emerging infectious disease. HME was first described in 1986, HGE in 1993, and E. *ewingii* first found in people in 1999. Very little is known about these diseases at this point; they are too new as human infectious agents. However incidences of infection are increasing each year in the United States and the disease has also spread to Europe. In 2002, about 500 cases were reported to the Centers for Disease Control. It is generally accepted that infections are seriously underreported. Because it is so new the disease is generally unrecognized by health practitioners. Those infected with Lyme disease tend to be the ones who are also reported as being infected with either HME or HGE. The primary form of infection is through tick bite.

The symptoms can include: fever (90%), headache (85%), myalgia (70%), arthralgia (70%), malaise (70%), thrombocytopenia (68%), leukopenia (60%), hyponatremia (40%), nausea (40%), vomiting (40%), enlarged liver and spleen (30%), mental confusion (20%), skin rash (10%), photophobia, anorexia, systolic murmur, conjunctivitis, strawberry tongue, pharyngitis, genital or oral ulcers, and abnormal gait. Diagnostic testing can be problematical unless the physician is knowledgeable about the disease. Generally, in Lyme disease it should be suspected and tested for. Treatment is generally with doxycycline.

However, treatment failures have occurred even at high doses. Rifampin seems to help in previous treatment failures if added to doxycycline.

Coinfection with ehrliciosis organisms is increasing. Testing has found coinfection with HGE in about 8% of at-risk populations in Italy and about the same amount in Wisconsin (U.S.). The two forms, HGE and HME, seem to settle into specific areas, specializing in certain populations. HGE is endemic in the Wisconsin/Minnesota area and HME along the eastern seaboard of the United States. Coinfection with borrelia and ehrliciosis organisms in rodent and tick populations has also been found in California, Colorado, Bulgaria, Germany, China, and Slovakia.

As with babesia, coinfection with ehrlichiosis organisms during Lyme infection increases the intensity of symptoms such as fever, chills, and dyspnea. Studies have found that mouse and rat immune responses are altered during confection with both Lyme and ehrlichia, pathogen burden is higher, and the severity of arthritic symptoms is greatly increased. Coinfection synergizes

> **TREATMENT OF EHRLICHIA COINFECTION**
>
> Tincture of Colchicum (autumn crocus): 20 drops daily for seven days.
>
> Astragalus capsules: 1,000-2,000 mg 3x daily for 30-60 days (see core protocol).

to suppress splenic Interleukin-2 (IL-2) production, to increase IL-4 production, and decrease Interferon gamma (IFN-gamma) production. This occurs at much greater levels than with either organism alone. Coinfection enhances expansion of splenic T cells, CD4+ lymphocytes and B cells, while decreasing CD8+ T cells.

Ehrlichia organisms have been found to be very susceptible to gamma interferon levels in the body. The best herb for stimulating gamma interferon is astragalus, which is why it is included in the protocol for ehrlichiosis infection.

AUTUMN CROCUS (*Colchicum autumnale*)

Common names: English: crocus, meadow saffron, naked ladies; colchico (Italian); colchique (France); and in Ayurvedic practice— surijan-i-talkh.

Family: Lily

Parts used: The bulb (aka corm) and seeds though the flowers have also
been used and are official in the German pharmacopoeia.

Habitat and Collection: The plant is native to southern, western, and
central Europe, and grows east to the banks of the Black Sea in
Georgia. It is cultivated heavily throughout the world. Related species
are common in India, China, and North Africa. The bulb is gathered
in early summer, the seeds in late summer or early fall.

Constituents: Acetyl dimethylcolchicine, demethylcolchicine, des-
methyldeacetylcolchicine, demethylbetalumicolchicine, demethyl-
gammalumichochicine, demethylcolchicine, desmethylcolchicine,
methylcolchicine, methoxysalicylic acid, alphalumicolchicine, apigenin, autumnaline, benzoic acid, beta-lumicolchicine, chelidonic
acid, coldhamine, colchicene, colchicerine, colchicine, colchifoling,
demecolcene, demecolcine, gamma-lumicolchicine, n-acetyldemecol-
cine, salicylic acid, and a bunch of other colchicine-type compounds.

Primarily of interest is the alkaloid colchicine. The seeds contain
about 0.4%, the bulb a bit less 0.35%, the fresh flowers vary considerably from 0.01%-0.08% while the dried flowers can contain up to 2%.
The leaves contain much less. Two and one-half grams of seeds contain about 10 mg of colchicine. The toxic dose of the pure constituent
colchicine runs from 5-7 mg (from hospital toxicity reports). Toxic
dose of colchicine in a whole-herb tincture is 8 mg (as per the
German Commission E Monographs).

Numerous members of the lily family contain colchicine. It is
seemingly a prevalent chemical among them, mostly found in the
bulbs. Inept laboratory analysis in two instances found colchicine in
ginkgo and echinacea but it is not really there.

Medicinal actions: Now primarily used for gout, arthritis, inflammation of the skin and joints, and treatment of familial Mediterranean
fever. It is increasingly being tested in American medical practice for
use in cases of recalcitrant constipation. It is a powerful anticonstipa-
tion agent. Colchicine inhibits parasitic invasion into erythrocytes
and has been used to treat malaria.

Colchicine is an extremely potent chemical and has been used for a great variety of conditions. It has been found effective against HIV and as an antibacterial against a number of organisms. It is considered to be anticirrhotic, antileukemic, antimeningitic, antipericarditic, antirheumatic, antithrombocytopenic, a powerful antimitotic, and a potent antitumor agent (breast, colon, and lung). It has historically been used for such things as fevers (specifically recurrent febrile diseases), bronchitis, and convulsions.

Functions in Lyme disease: Antibacterial for ehrlichia coinfection. Potent antiarthritic and anti-inflammatory.

About autumn crocus: The herb has been used for at least three thousand years throughout the Mediterranean region for gout and rheumatism. Its emergence as an important member of the herbal apothecary occurred during the great Islamic renaissance nearly twelve hundred years ago, where it's then-common name translates as "the soul of the joints." It was in common use among the ancient Greeks and Romans and has been an official part of western botanic practice for centuries. The person primarily responsible for spreading its use in the western world for the treatment of gout and arthritis was Jacob Psychristus, the fifth-century Byzantine physician.

Ayurveda: A related species, *Colchicum luteum*, also containing colchicum, has been used in India for millennia for gout, rheumatism, and diseases of the liver and spleen.

Traditional Chinese medicine: The herb has been used in China for millennia, mostly for similar conditions.

Western botanic practice: The herb has been a regular part of western botanic practice for centuries, moving through ancient Greek and Roman cultures and thence into emerging European cultures. The American Eclectic physicians used it, and it is still official in the German pharmacopoeia and listed in the German Commission E monographs.

Specific indications in Eclectic practice were: Gout, gouty diathesis, rheumatism, tearing pain that is aggravated by heat, pain in the nerves, gouty headache with swelling of the joints, constipation, nervousness, sudden tearing pain up and down limbs without fever.

In current German practice, specific uses are for acute gout and familial Mediterranean fever. It is considered to be: anti-chemotactic, antiphlogistic, and an inhibitor of mitosis.

Scientific: Colchicum is specifically indicated in the treatment of ehrlichia infections in that its major constituent, colchicine is rapidly distributed to leukocytes—the same cells invaded by ehrlichia organisms. Concentration of colchicine in leukocytes is rapid and tends to exceed that in plasma. It can be detected in leukocytes for 9-10 days following the ingestion of a single dose of colchicine.

Colchicine normalizes abnormalities of lymphocyte and monocyte function and reverses abnormalities in neutrophil activity. It reduces increased migration of neutrophils into inflamed tissues, and increases superoxide scavenging activity.

Colchicine accumulates in the gastrointestinal wall, kidneys, liver, spleen, and in leukocytes. This is especially useful in treating HME-type ehrlichiosis in that infection with *Ehrlichia chafeensis* (the agent of human monocytic ehrlichiosis, HME) not only invades macrophages in the bloodstream, but also liver, spleen, and kidney macrophages.

The herb is specifically indicated for autoimmune inflammatory conditions: ankolysing spondylitis, rheumatoid arthritis, sarcoidosis, amyloidosis, Behcet's disease, familial Mediterranean fever, and so on. The action is broad. Behcet's disease is an chronic inflammatory condition of the blood vessels with secondary inflammation of synovia, skin, bowel, and brain/spinal cord. Familial Mediterranean fever (FMF) is a hereditary disease usually found in Armenians and Sephardic Jews. It presents as short, recurrent attacks of fever and pain in the abdomen, chest, or joints, and erythema. The herb and its constituent, colchicine, are specific for these kinds of conditions, and reliably reduce inflammation in many of the acute conditions (gout) or prevent acute attacks in others (FMF). Colchicine specifically inhibits the movement of neutrophils and macrophages into damaged tissues in autoimmune-inflammatory conditions. It has been found to have specific effects on interleukin-6 (IL-6), IL-8, tumor necrosis factor-alpha (TNF-alpha), and soluble E- and L-selectin levels in inflammatory conditions.

In gout, colchicine inhibits the deposit of uric acid crystals in tissues and stops the inflammatory process that is occurring. It also inhibits microtubule formation assembly in a number of different cells, including leukocytes. In essence, colchicine binds to and inhibits the polymerization of tubulin, which plays an essential role in cellular division. This is one of the reasons it is so potent in cancer treatment (and also why it is not recommended during pregnancy). This microtubule depolymerization action is also what inhibits the proliferation of ehrlichia organisms.

Colchicine spreads rapidly throughout the body within three to five minutes of ingestion. In healthy individuals, 10%-15% of the colchicine is eliminated from the body daily, primarily in urine, bile, and feces. In the ill a bit less is excreted—8%-10%. These elimination rates need to be kept in mind during dosing.

Medline lists 251 clinical trials with colchicine, either alone or in combination therapy. *In vivo* and *in vitro* studies are even more numerous. In spite of three thousand years of practitioner use and its current place as a part of German, Ayurvedic, and Chinese practice, no clinical trials (that I can find) have been conducted with use of the whole herb. A few *in vitro* studies do exist, however, showing that extracts of the whole herb stimulate the activity of human leukocytes and lymphocytes.

In vivo tests have found colchicine to be as effective as silymarin in the treatment of chronic carbon tetrachloride liver damage in rats. Colchicine and silymarin both completely prevented all changes observed in the livers of CCl4-treated rats. Human trials of the constituent in the treatment of active liver disease have been mixed; outcomes were not good in active hepatitis C and B infections. It has shown some good results in the treatment of biliary cirrhosis and liver fibrosis and excellent results in the treatment of ascites. Ascitic fluid disappeared entirely from 73% of those taking colchicine without the use of diuretics. Recurrence was about 48% among colchicine users versus 83% among those who used diuretics.

Clinical trials have found colchicine to be effective for such condition as: recurrent acute idiopathic pericarditis, Behcet's disease, familial Mediterranean fever, gout, osteoarthritis, recurrent aphthous stomatis, Peyronie's disease (codosed with vitamin E), chronic bulbous dermatosis, cutaneous leukocytoclastic vasculitis, mixed cryoglobulinemia, IgE-mediated early and late-airway reactions, as a preventative for postpericardiotomy syndrome, severe chronic constipation, low back pain (IM injection), and topically in a cream for actinic keratoses.

Both *in vivo* and *in vitro* studies have found the constituent to be active against *Ehrlichia risticii*. One human study, treating infections by the organism *Anaplasma phagocytophila* (formerly *Ehrlichia phagocytophilia*) found colchicine effective.

Dosage: *Please read carefully.* Although serious side effects from use of the herb are exceptionally uncommon (in contrast to the isolated constituent, colchicine), this herb is potentially very toxic and should be used with caution and under the supervision of a knowledgeable practitioner. The sale of the tincture is regulated in some states (e.g. New Jersey) as a schedule-B substance. Colchicine accumulates in the system, and continual dosing can produce toxic impacts over time even if the dose remains low. The isolated constituent, colchicine, is considerably more toxic than the herb itself and most toxicity studies are on that isolated chemical. Generally, with intelligent use, the herb can be utilized as safely as it is in Germany in standard botanical practice.

German Commission E Monograph dosage with the tincture of bulb, seeds, or flower is:

"For acute attack [of gout], an initial dose corresponding to 1 mg colchicine, followed by 0.5-1.5 mg every 1-2 hours until pain subsides. Total daily dosage must not surpass 8 mg colchicine.

"For familial Mediterranean fever, prophylactic and therapeutic purposes, dosage corresponding to 0.5-1.5 mg of colchicine."

Eclectic dosage was "tincture of root 10-60 drops, tincture of seed 10-40 drops."

On average, a drop of seed tincture will contain about 60 micrograms of colchicine, and the root about the same although the roots were considered to be less potent in Eclectic practice. Prophylactic dosage is considered to be around 600 mcg or 10 drops of tincture.

Acute condition dose is then 30 drops of tincture (Commission E) containing about 1.8 mg colchicine (60 drops per teaspoon, 360 drops per ounce).

For ehrlichiosis: 20 drops (2.5 ml) tincture daily for seven days. Repeat in 10 days if necessary.

Side effects: *Please read carefully.* There are a number of side effects from use of the herb, primarily loose stools and diarrhea at larger doses. (Colchicine is excellent for constipation as the clinical trials have shown.) The German Commission E Monographs list the following as potential side effects from using herbal preparations of the plant: diarrhea, nausea, vomiting, abdominal pain, leukopenia. With extended use: skin alterations, agranulocytosis, aplastic anemia, myopathy, alopecia.

- **In the event of side effects reduce dose or discontinue use of the herb.**
- Only one report exists (that I can find) on toxic overdose with an herbal preparation of autumn crocus and that from the nineteenth century—someone drank a lot of crocus wine. There are, however, deaths every year from people who mistake the plant for something else (usually garlic or onion) and eat the root or leaves. Fatalities in healing practice all occur from use of pharmaceutical preparations of colchicine prescribed by physicians. It is much more potent, and dangerous, than the whole plant preparation.

Tincture preparation: Vinegar tincture: An acetic or vinegar tincture is prepared by macerating one and one-half ounces of the dried bulb or seeds in 12 ounces of "the strongest" vinegar for 14 days. Press and strain. Dose: 10-60 drops (King's American Dispensatory).

Alcohol tincture: 1:5, 70% alcohol, 30% water. Colchicine is easily soluble in both water and alcohol. One ounce of seeds in five ounces of liquid will give about 110 mg of colchicine which gives about 60 mcg per drop.

Standardized tincture: From about 1880, as chemistry became more sophisticated as a science, the amount of colchicine in the tinctures were controlled by the pharmacists preparing them. The tinctures were prepared using 1000 grams of dried and powdered root, two parts alcohol and one part water. The extract was assayed and standardized to provide 0.35 grams of colchicine per 100 ml of tincture (U.S. National Formulary, 1916). Regrettably, pharmacists are no longer trained to do this; mostly, they put pills from large containers into smaller ones.

While the amount of colchicine is less controlled in the vinegar and non-formulary tinctures, they did work well for several millennia prior to the development of chemical assay techniques. Again, the herb should be used with intelligent caution.

Contraindications: Not to be used in pregnancy as it causes fetal abnormality. Not to be taken when breast feeding as colchicine transmits easily through breast milk. Not to be used in those with abnormal renal and hepatic function, especially in those with liver and kidney impairment. May impair healing and increase infection from dental surgery. Should be used with extreme caution in active alcoholism due to its impacts on liver and GI tract.

Herb/drug interactions: Short-term use of colchicum is fine. However, long-term use has shown a number of herb/drug interactions that should be carefully monitored. Generally, long-term use is not indicated in the treatment of ehrlichia infections.

Nonsteroidal anti-inflamatories should not be used with the herb as they can increase the risk of gastrointestinal ulceration. May increase the anticoagulation action of blood-thinning medications (anticoagulants, heparin, thrombolytic agents, platelet aggregation inhibitors, and so on). Not to be used with blood dyscrasia-causing medications. May interfere with the absorption of vitamin B-12.

BARTONELLA

Bartonella are gram-negative, aerobic bacteria and are considered emerging pathogens. Even though one form of bartonellosis was recognized as early as 1889 (cat-scratch disease) and another in World War I (trench fever), the causative organisms were not identified until the late twentieth century.

In 1992, *Rochalimaea henselae* was identified as the causative organism of cat-scratch disease. Its Latin name was recently changed to *Bartonella henselae*. Like borrelia organisms, bartonella organisms are considered to be fastidious. That is, they are hard to grow in the laboratory. This has impeded research on the organisms and the diseases they cause.

> **TREATMENT OF BARTONELLA COINFECTION**
>
> *Polygonum cuspidatum* tablets: 3-4, 4x daily.
>
> Boneset tea: 3-4x daily
>
> Red root tincture (with lymph, spleen, or liver inflammation): 30-90 drops to 4x daily

At this point, there are four bartonella species that are considered to be factors in human disease. Emerging research is, however, indicating that this number is going to rise. *Bartonella quintana* causes trench fever, first recognized in WWI. It is transmitted by lice and occurs mostly among the homeless. *B. henselae*, or cat-scratch disease, is the organism usually found as a coninfectious agent with Lyme disease. *B. bacilliformis* is transmitted by sand flies that live at higher elevations in the Andes. It causes Oroya fever and is the most severe form of bartonellosis. *B. elizabethae* is a newly discovered bartonella organism that causes endocarditis.

A number of new and unique bartonella organisms have recently been found in biting flies and ticks in California. The species found in the ticks were unusual and similar, although not identical, to *B. henselae, B. quintana, B. washoensis*, and *B. vinsonii*. These latter-two species usually cause infections in animals. Bartonella species appear to be undergoing subtle and rapid genomic alterations much like borrelia spirochetes. An unusual bartonella variant was also found in ticks and mice in Martha's Vineyard in 1998—again, similar to but not the same as two bartonella organisms known for animal infections: *B. vinsonii* and *B. grahamii*. At least two *B. henselae* genotypes have been identified. There does not seem to be a species wall with respect to bartonella transmission.

Concurrent bartonella infections have been found, and are increasingly being found, in Lyme disease. And as with other coinfectious agents, the severity of each disease is increased, especially if there is central-nervous-system involvement.

The general symptoms of bartonella infection are: swollen lymph glands (80%), low-grade fever (50-70%), malaise and fatigue (70%), enlarged spleen (11%), anorexia (15%), headache (14%), pharyngitis (8%), rash (5%), conjunctivitis (6%), CNS involvement (2%), sore muscles and joints (arthritis, synovitis, etc), and aching or painful bones. With coinfection, these symptoms are more common and severe.

Bartonella organisms tend to be species specific; that is, they specialize in who they infect. Once adapted to a particular species, they present a different pathology than when unadapted.

In all cases they quickly move into endothelial tissue. However, once adapted to a new species, they periodically move from that location into red blood cells. This creates a periodically recurring malaria-like (or babesiosis-like) disease. In non-adapted species, the disease is generally less severe and resolves on its own (e.g., cat-scratch disease).

Bartonella henselae bacteria are in the process of establishing an adaptive relationship with human beings, something that has already occurred with both *B. quintana* and *B. bacilliformis.*

In animal hosts, the bacteria enter the body through a vector such as a flea, biting fly, or tick and colonize the endothelial cells, periodically releasing bacteria that infect red blood cells. This allows vectors such as ticks to uptake the organism during feeding and spread it into new animals. Red blood-cell infection can be very high—anemia is one symptom during active infection and can be quite serious. Because long-term adaptation has not yet occurred with *B. henselae* in human beings, red blood-cell infection tends to be low.

The bacteria also infect macrophages, stimulating a release of proinflammatory cytokines—tumor necrosis factor alpha, interleukin IB, and IL-6. *In vitro* studies have found that stimulating macrophages with interferon gamma significantly increases macrophage bactericidal action against bartonella organisms and thus decreases the levels of infected macrophages. Spleen and liver involvement is usually high during infection; mild spleen inflammation is common.

Infection in a non-reservoir host, such as people, by *B. henselae* leads to five primary disease manifestations: cat-scratch disease, fever with bacteremia, endocarditis, bacillary angiomatosis, or peliosis hepatitis. The severity, or even the emergence, of these manifestations depends on how strong the immune system is. Coinfection with Lyme reduces immune strength, increasing the impacts of the disease. Fever with bacteremia is very common.

The bacteria are intracellular organisms. That is, they live inside the cells. They have a particular affinity for endothelial cells where they exhibit potent angiogenesis-stimulating actions. In immunocompromised people, such as those with AIDS, this angiogenesis stimulation is severe and often causes proliferative vascular tumors. The organisms stimulate neovascularization in the small blood vessels causing, in some instances, bacillary angiomatosis, bacillary splenitis, and/or peliosis hepatitis. They are good at avoiding host-immune responses (phagocytosis) and become intravascularly persistent. The organisms significantly impact endothelial cell function. Primary endothelial impacts are cell invasion, proinflammatory activation, suppression of apoptosis, and simulation of proliferation. The bacteria always cause (to greater or lesser degrees of severity) proliferation of microvascular endothelial cells and neovascularization (angiogenesis).

Bacillary angiomatosis and bacillary splenitis have been found, however, not only in immunocompromised people but also in immunocompetent adults, indicating that these complications of bartonella infection are potentially more common and widespread than currently believed. Testing for bartonella infection in those conditions has not been routine.

There is increasing evidence that bartonella organisms also infect bone marrow in addition to endothelial cells. While their main reservoir in the body is the endothelial cells, infection of bone marrow is important to the pathogenesis of the disease. The symptoms of bone infection are generally mild to nonexistent in *B. henselae* infection. They are much more severe with *B. quintana* (trench fever), which causes extreme pain in the shins.

In bone marrow, mature erythroblasts are produced in structures called erythroblastic islands. When mature, these move across the endothelial barrier into circulation in the blood. Erythroid cells coexpress two potent angiogenic factors: vascular endothelial growth factor (VEGF) and placental growth factor. Bartonella bacteria enter bone marrow, colonize erythroblastic islands (composed of a central macrophage surrounded by maturing erythroblasts) and stimulate the release of VEGF. VEGF stimulates the migration and permeability of endothelial cells and the migration of monocytes.

VEGF is a potent endothelial cell mitogen and key regulator of both physiologic and pathologic angiogenesis. Bartonella bacteria use VEGF to control and maximize their intrusion into endothelial cells. The more immunocompromised a person is the greater the negative effects this bacteria-stimulated VEGF proliferation will be.

Inflammation in endothelial cells occurs because bartonella bacteria induce the expression of nuclear-factor kappa B (NF-kB) and its upregulation of adhesion molecules in infected endothelial cells. During this kind of inflammatory process, neutrophils "roll over" (PMN rolling) the bacterial-stimulated endothelium, then adhere to its surface in an attempt to deal with the infection. Bartonella infections are accompanied by significantly increased PMN rolling and adhesion. Cell-adhesion factors, E-selectin and ICAM-1 (intracellular adhesion molecule-1) are strongly upregulated by bartonella infection. The induction of these adhesion molecules is stimulated by NF-kB activation. The outer-protein membrane coat of the bacteria stimulate this process. This inflammatory dynamic causes extravasation or leakage in the endothelial tissues, facilitating penetration of the organism into the cells.

During this process, bartonella bacteria initiate massive rearrangements of the actin cytoskeleton which result in the formation of bacterial aggregates on the surface of endothelial cells. Basically, the bacteria attach to the cell membrane and then clump together on the cellular surface. This aggregate—the invasome—is taken into the interior of the cell. The process is facilitated by the upregulation of ICAM-1 and another compound cortical F-actin. The bacteria then release substances that inhibit apoptic cell death and cytostatic and cytotoxic cell activity that could interfere with the bacteria's mitogenic activity. The bacteria then begin to release substances that stimulate the proliferation of endothelial cells, eventually causing the formation of new blood vessels. Endothelial engulfment allows the bacteria to reproduce (it's a slow grower) relatively protected from the host immune response. It replicates within the engulfed invasome and periodically releases bacteria into the bloodstream where, in adapted hosts, red blood cells are infected and then picked up by ticks or biting flies and passed onto other animals.

During chronic infection, host-immune defenses are compromised, and bacterial phagocytosis is impaired. There is a sustained decrease in CD8+ lymphocytes, increased CD4+ T cells and impaired antigen presentation to helper T cells. The bacteria actively suppresses immune response in chronic infection.

Twenty-four thousand bartonella cases a year are reported, although that is believed to be a low indication of actual infection rates. Diagnosis of the disease is often poor due to its emerging nature and lack of recognition among physicians.

Tests for bartonella have been found to be only about 85% effective. Treatment response is mixed. Review articles have been unclear as to the best treatment and some researchers note (Fournier, 1998) that "CSD [*Bartonella henselae*] typically does not respond to antibiotic therapy. Only the aminoglycosides, mainly gentamicin, were reported as effective in patients suffering suppurative complications. A few reports indicate that ciprofloxacin, rifampin, and trimethoprim-sulfamethoxazole may be active." The Canadian Lyme Disease Foundation comments that "In the co-infected Lyme patient, eradication may be difficult." Articles by specialists on the treatment of this disease rarely indicate the same pharmaceuticals for the condition or the same length of time that dosage should be instituted, illustrating both the newness of the disease and confusion about its exact pathogenesis and treatment. The most recent studies seem to indicate that long-term antibiotic treatment with azithromycin, doxycycline, and rifampin is the most effective approach. Colchicine has been specifically tested against bartonella and is ineffective.

Nonantibiotic therapies should emphasize the use of *Polygonum cuspidatum* to counteract the angiogenesis actions of the organisms, boneset to stimulate immune response, and red root to clear the lymph system (if needed). These may be used along with antibiotic treatment with good effect. *Stephania* should be considered as a secondary approach.

In brief, polygonum (resveratrol) will inhibit NF-kB upregulation, stopping the inflammatory response that is so important for endothelial penetration by bartonella organisms. It is also an angiogenesis modulator and will stop the angiogenesis-stimulating action of the bacteria. It is a potent inhibitor of vascular endothelial growth factor, which is stimulated by the bacteria. The plant will strongly protect the body against the proliferation of microvascular endothelial cells and neovascularization (angiogenesis). It will also address most of the symptoms of bartonella infection and protect the heart from inflammation. It is, as well, a strong antibacterial and a modulator of immune response during infections. Please see the whole-plant listing in the Core Protocol section.

CHAPTER SIX

Prevention of Lyme
and Initial Treatment
for Rash or Tickbite

This chapter outlines an herbal protocol designed to prevent or lessen the impacts of Lyme-disease infection, and another to begin immediately if you discover the typical Lyme rash or an attached tick. Immediately using the protocol once you discover the Lyme rash will reduce the severity of the disease and significantly enhance outcomes, whether you use herbs or antibiotics or both.

Of the substances listed below, the borrelia nosode will initiate a mild vaccine-like action, the andrographis will potentiate your immune system and maintain an antispirochetal activity in your body, and the cat's claw will enhance immune function. These will help prevent infection. If you should become infected in spite of these precautions, the herbs you have been using will have stimulated your immune system to be more active, and your CD57 white blood-cell count will be high. This will help reduce the severity of the infection, increase your body's ability to get rid of the infection during treatment, and lessen the chance of the disease becoming chronic.

ASTRAGALUS

Studies with tick-borne infection in mice found that if levels of interferon gamma and interleukin 2 were high in the animals, infection by

FOR PREVENTION IF YOU LIVE IN A LYME-ENDEMIC AREA:

Astragalus herb, all year:
1,000 mg daily

FOR PREVENTION AT THE BEGINNING OF THE TICK SEASON TAKE:

Homeopathic borrelia nosode 30C: 3x daily for three days.

Andrographis (400 mg): 1 capsule 3x daily throughout the season.

Cat's claw (500 mg): 2 capsules 3x daily throughout the season.

(See Core Protocol, chapter two for contraindications and side effects)

AT THE FIRST SIGN OF BULL'S-EYE RASH (EM) OR EMBEDDED TICK:

For rash, homeopathic apis 30C: 3x daily for three days

For tickbite, homeopathic ledum 1M: 3x daily for three days.

Begin core protocol for Lyme disease

Eleuthero tincture: 1 tsp 3x daily for 30-60 days

(See chapter four for further Eleuthero information)

borrelia spirochetes was much lower than otherwise. The reduction of these components, especially interleukin-2, is stimulated through components in the tick saliva. Keeping levels high will significantly reduce the likelihood of infection. Astragalus is a powerful immune-tonic herb. In-depth studies in people and in animals have found that it stimulates the production of both interleukin-2 and interferon gamma. The herb should be taken year-round if you live in a Lyme-endemic area.

HOMEOPATHIC BORRELIA NOSODE

Homeopaths, although few know it, pioneered the concept of vaccinations through the use of nosodes. Nosodes are exceptionally weak forms of the kinds of vaccinations that were originally created for things like smallpox and they are made in much the same manner. They are very dilute (as are all homeopathic medicines) solutions and their production is regulated by the FDA. Unlike the vaccine for Lyme disease, there are no reports of side effects from the use of the borrelia nosode. Studies have found, however, that nosodes are much weaker in their protective effects than vaccines, although the same studies show they are significantly better than nothing at all.

Oddly enough, even though they do provide some degree of protection from infection, examination has shown that nosodes do not increase antibodies in those who take them as a preventative for disease.

There have not been a great many clinical studies on the effectiveness of nosodes, but there have been a few.

One study in 1974 examined the occurrence of meningitis in 18,640 children who received a single dose of meningococcinum nosode (10C, single dose) during an epidemic in Brazil. Only four developed meningitis (0.02%). Meningitis occurrence in the control group of 6,340 children who did not receive the nosode was 0.5%. Thirty-two in that group of children became ill.

Comparisons of a tularemia nosode against a standard vaccine in mice showed that the nosode did, in fact, offer protection. While the vaccines conferred 100% immunity, the nosode conferred 22% immunity (compared to 0% in the untreated mice). The nosode significantly increased the life span in the other 78% of mice who were not protected from infection.

Clinical research on an intestinal dysentery nosode over a 30-year period of time showed that it, too, provided protection against infection. And a study of 50,000 children who took a polio nosode in the 1950s found that the incidence of polio was below that of untreated children— only one child became infected and that was a nonparalytic form.

Dosage: Homeopathic borrelia nosode 30C: 3x daily for three days.

Steven Tobin (see homeopathic ledum) recommends the following dosage for Lyme for a vaccine-like prevention in dogs: Borrelia nosode 60C, one dose daily for one week, then one dose per week for one month, then one dose every six months.

Side effects and contraindications: None known.

HOMEOPATHIC APIS AND LEDUM

Homeopathic medicines are, like nosodes, regulated by the FDA. They are manufactured under strict guidelines for purity and production. Homeopathic medicines are exceptionally weak as they are diluted considerably before sale. There has been a tremendous antipathy between medical doctors and homeopaths in the United States for at least 150 years. It shows no signs of abating.

There have been few clinical studies on homeopathic preparations in the treatment of disease, although more are occurring each year. Significantly, they are beginning to show that, as homeopathic practitioners have insisted, there is something in what they do.

In some circumstances, homeopathic medicines are exceptionally effective in the treatment of disease. There has been some degree of clinical success in the use of homeopathic medicines for the treatment of Lyme disease. There have been no clinical studies.

Homeopathic apis is made from honey-bee venom and has been used for over 150 years in the homeopathic treatment of diseases like hives and psoriasis, situations characterized by rashes, swellings, redness, and inflammation in the skin. Generally, hot, burning, inflamed conditions of any sort. Homeopaths have reported some good success with homeopathic apis in the treatment of Lyme disease, especially at onset or with long-term chronic Lyme.

Homeopathic ledum, made from the plant *Ledum palustre* (aka marsh rosemary), is the primary preparation used by homeopaths for treating bites and stings from insects. Secondarily, it is used for skin rashes like those caused by poison oak and poison ivy. It is often used as a preventive after exposure but before actual infection occurs. The primary interest in homeopathic ledum has come from the work of Steven Tobin, a veterinarian who works in an area where Lyme is endemic. After treating over 500 dogs for Lyme disease, he commented that "Every animal treated this way has shown immediate improvement, whether they were only recently infected or have had the disease for years, treated or not with antibiotics. A number of pet owners, on seeing how well it cured their companions, took it themselves, with equally good results."

The general report from practitioners who have prescribed homeopathic ledum and people who have used it is, however, mixed. Most find that it sometimes helps but this is primarily when taken just after tick bite and before the disease becomes full blown.

Nevertheless, the remedy is inexpensive and without side effects, and it does sometimes help.

Dosages: At onset of rash, homeopathic apis 30C: 3x daily for three days. At discovery of tickbite, homeopathic ledum 1M: 3x daily for three days.

Side effects and contraindications: Do not use homeopathic apis if pregnant, otherwise none known.

For the use of non-homeopathic Apis in the treatment of Lyme disease: Please see the Articles listing at my website: www.gaianstudies.org.

CHAPTER SEVEN

The Lyme Protocol and Repertory Streamlined

🐝

LYME BORRELIOSIS

1.0 Prevention

in endemic areas—astragalus daily

at beginning of tick season—borrelia nosode

for duration of tick season—astragalus, andrographis, Uncaria

at tick bite—homeopathic ledum, core protocol (*Andrographis paniculata, Polygonum cuspidatum, Uncaria tomentosa, Astragalus*).

at appearance of rash—homeopathic apis, core protocol

1.1 Acute Onset

general—eleutherococcus, core protocol

1.2 Antispirochetals

Andrographis paniculata, Polygonum cuspidatum, Stephania tetrandra (or cepharantha), Anthriscus sylvestris, Apis, Bi-EDTA

1.3 Bell's Palsy

specific—stephania (tetrandra or cepharantha)

recalcitrant—stephania, acupuncture

supportive—vitamin B-12

1.4 Neuroborreliosis

reduction of inflammation—polygonum, stephania

neuroprotection—polygonum, stephania, smilax, huperzine A, zinc

supportive—astragalus, eleutherococcus

1.5 Lyme Neurotoxins

to inhibit production of/counteract—polygonum, selenium, zinc picinolate with copper, melatonin

1.6 Memory and Cognitive Dysfunction

general—polygonum, stephania, huperzine A, vinpocetine, L-acetylcarnetine, zinc

1.7 Depression

Swedish massage weekly, eleutherococcus

1.8 Eye Involvement (Ocularborreliosis)

specific—stephania

supportive—vinpocetine, vitamin C, zinc

1.9 Lyme Arthritis

general—polygonum, stephania, Dipsacus sylvestris, smilax, vitamin A

pain—curcumin/bromelain combination, harpagophytum, urtica, capsaicin (cream, topical)

collagen support—see 1.14

1.10 Dermatoborreliosis

erythema migrans—andrographis, polygonum, homeopathic apis, smilax

acrodermatitis chronica atropicans—pregnenolone, andrographis, polygonum, apis, vitamin C, smilax

1.11 Muscle Twitches, Tingling/Crawling Sensations

general—vitamins B-12, B-6, Folic acid, magnesium

1.12 Lyme Carditis

with angina—polygonum, stephania, astragalus, crataegus, Amni visnaga

with arrhythmia—stephania, crataegus

with palpitations—polygonum, astragalus

with shortness of breath—polygonum, astragalus

1.13 Immune Modulation

   low immune function—astragalus, andrographis, uncaria, eleutherococcus, smilax

   raise CD57 count—uncaria, bromelain, vitamin E

   enhance CD4+, balance CD4/CD8 ratio—polygonum, astragalus

   early stage stimulation—polygonum, astragalus, eleutherococcus

   low Th1 at initial infection—astragalus

   high Th1, late stage—stephania

   modulate hyperimmune response in late stage Lyme—stephania

   modulate HLA-DR expression—stephania, uncaria, astragalus

1.14 Lyme Infection, Collagen Tissues Support

   general—pregnenolone, zinc, copper, silicon, DHEA, alpha lipoic
acid, selenium, glucosamine sulfate, vitamin B complex, vitamin C,
vitamin E

1.15 Headaches

   general—andrographis, vinpocetine, polygonum, stephania

1.16 Chronic Fatigue

   general—eleutherococcus, andrographis, astragalus, Swedish massage weekly

   acute—eleutherococcus (Russian formulation)

1.17 Muscle Weakness

   general—pinus (pollen), Aralia naudicaulis, Panax quinquefolius—
combination tincture.

1.18 Swollen Lymph Nodes or Sluggish Lymph

   general—ceanothus, Phytolacca decandra, Swedish massage weekly

1.19 Post Lyme Disease Syndrome

   with hypoperfusion—ginkgo

   with memory deficits—huperzine A, vinpocetine

   with weakness and fatigue—eleutherococcus

1.20 Sluggish Thyroid

   general—eleutherococcus

   as tonic—raphanus (radish, black or daikon), Fucus vesiculosus

1.21 Babesia Coinfection

   specific—artemisinin

   supportive—ceanothus

   for chills/fever/sweats—Eupatorium perfoliatum

1.22 Ehrlichia Coinfection

specific—colchicum

supportive—astragalus

1.23 Bartonella Coinfection

specific—polygonum

to clear detritus—ceanothus

for chills/fever/sweats—Eupatorium perfoliatum

1.24 For Reducing Herxheimer Reactions

smilax, Polygonum cuspidatum

1.25 For Candida Overgrowth from Antibiotics

caprylic acid, undecenoic acid, thymic Formula, molybdenum picinolate.

1.26 To Maintain Bowel Health While on Antibiotics

Probiotic 8 (PB8) or equivalent

RESOURCES

Lyme Literate Physicians and/or Referrals:

1. Lyme Disease Association
   www.lymediseaseassociation.org
   888-366-6611

2. kimuffleman@hotmail.com
   (suggested by www.Ilads.com)

3. Tedde Rinker, D. O.
   2055 Woodside Road, Suite 160
   Redwood City, CA 94061
   650-367-1988
   www.stress-medicine.com

3. Dr. Steven Harris, M.D.
   Pacific Frontier Medical, Inc.
   570 Price Avenue, Suite 200
   Redwood City, CA 94063
   T: (650) 474-2130

4. Dr. Jeffrey Wulfman, M.D.
   61 Court Drive
   Brandon, VT 05733
   (802) 247-3756 or
   (802) 247-3755

Chinese Medicine Practitioners:

1. Zhang Clinic
   420 Lexington Avenue
   New York, NY 10170
   212-573-9584

2. Tim Scott, L. Ac.
   62 Elliot Street
   Brattleboro, VT 05301
   802-251-0888 (NOTE: Tim is exceptionally familiar with the protocol in this book)

3. Sarah Gardner, L. Ac.
   14720 107th Way
   Vashon, WA 98070
   206-940-8802

I can no longer recommend Dierdre O'Connor
or anyone on staff at Natura Medica in Mystic, CT.
I regret any inconvenience this has caused or may
cause anyone.

Herbalists and/or Herbalist Referrals:
Julie McIntyre
8 Pioneer Road
Silver City, NM 88061
julie@gaianstudies.org
575-538-5498
(NOTE: Julie is exceptionally familiar with the protocol in this book)

Kathleen Maier
Sacred Plant Traditions
The Glass Building
313 Second Street, Suite 211
Charlottesville, VA 22902
434-295-3820
www.sacredplanttraditions.com

Northeast Herbal Association
P.O.Box 103
Manchaug, MA 01526
neha@northeastherbal.org

American Herbalists Guild
1931 Gaddis Road
Canton, GA 30115
770-751-6021
ahgoffice@earthlink.net
www.americanherbalistsguild.com

Testing and Diagnosis

Joseph Burrascano, M.D. *Diagnostic Hints and Treatment Guidelines for Lyme and Other Tick Borne Illnesses*, 14th Edition, November 2002. www.ilads.org/burrascano_1102.html. Accessed 12/17/2004. **Highly recommended.**

Bowen Research
Rapid Identification of Borrelia burgdorferi (RIBb) test
38541 US HWY 19N
Palm Harbor, FL 34684
727-937-9077
www.bowen.org

IgeneX
Lyme Dot Immunoassay (LDA)
797 San Antonio Road
Palo Alto, CA 94303
800-832-3200
www.igenex.com
Also tests for babesia and ehrlichia

Stricker NK Panel CD-57 test
LabCorp: www.labcorp.com
510-635-4555
LabCorp purchased IDL, the company that originally developed this test. LabCorp is a monster corporation and this test, while still offered by the company, is relatively unknown to them and not listed on their Web site. LabCorp has numerous collection sites around the country. The one nearest you can be found by searching their Web site. Your physician will need to know the codes used by LabCorp for them to provide the test. Diagnosis: ICD-9 for Lyme: 088.81. Test procedure code and description: Test ID# 32103-5, Stricker NK Panel CD-57. More information on the specifics of this test and how your physician should proceed can be found at www.anapsid.org/lyme/strickerpanel.html (accessed 2/1/05). The

Stricker panel tests for white blood cells, lymphocytes, % T cells
(CD3+), % NK Subset (CD57+/CD8), %CD8+/CD57+, total lympho-
cytes, total T cells (Cd3), total CD8+/CD57+, total NK subset
(CD57+/CD8+).

HERBAL SOURCES:
General:
Woodland Essence
P.O. Box 206
Cold Brook, NY 13324
315-845-1515
www.woodlandessence.com

Japanese Knotweed (Polygonum cuspidatum):
Bulk Polygonum:
1st Chinese herbs
5018 View Ridge Drive
Olympia, WA 98501
888-842-2049 (toll free)
www.1stchineseherbs.com

Wildcrafted Bulk Polygonum:
Woodland Essence
P.O.Box 206
Cold Brook, NY 13324
315-845-1515
www.woodlandessence.com

Tablet Form:
Source Naturals Resveratrol contains 500 mg of Polygonum cuspidatum and resveratrols, standardized to 8%, and 10 mg resveratrol
(piceid, resveratrol glucoside) www.myvitanet.com
800-807-8080

Stephania Root (*Stephania tetrandra*):
1st Chinese herbs
5018 view Ridge Drive
Olympia, WA 98501
888-842-2049 (toll free)
www.1stchineseherbs.com
(best price)

Yan Jing Supply
1441 York Street
Denver, CO 80206
866.837.1346
www.yanjingsupply.com
(sold by the gram—0.07 per gm)

Pure Land Ethnobotanicals
2701 University Ave, PMB 463
Madison, WI 53705
info@ethnobotanicals.com
(Expensive)

Mayway Corporation
1338 Mandela parkway
Oakland, CA 94607
info@mayway.com
800.262.9929
(Licensed practitioners only)

Stephania tincture is available from:
www.biopureus.com
www.nihadc.com

SUPPLEMENTS:

Hardbody Nutrition
800-378-6787
www.hardbodynutrition.com
Best site for price on HerbPharm eleuthero. Generally will beat any
other outlet's prices by 5% on anything they carry.

Wholesale Nutrition
P.O.Box 3345
Saratoga, CA 95070
800-325-2664
408-871-9519
www.nutri.com
Best source for effervescent vitamin C and many supplements. NOTE:
With this company it is better to rely on phone orders only, and not go
through the internet site, which is not really set up to take orders.
(Your order will never come if you send it via email.)

Seacoast Natural Foods
800-555-6792
www.seacoastvitamins.com
A good general source for many herbs and supplements.

REFERENCES

LYME BORRELIOSIS:

Alban, P. et al. Serum-starvation-induced changes in protein synthesis and morphology of Borrelia burgdorferi, *Microbiology* 2000;146 (Pt 1):119-27.

Anonymous. Persistence or Relapse of Lyme Disease Despite "appropriate" or "Conventional" Antibiotic Therapy: A Bibliography with Highlighted Full Abstracts. www.geocities.com/HotSprings/Oasis/6455/persistence-special-abstracts.html. Accessed 12/8/2004.

————. Reasons for the Survival and Persistence of Lyme Disease Bacteria (cystic forms, blebs, L-forms, etc.): A bibliography with highlighted full abstracts. www.geocities.com/HotSprings/Oasis.6455.persistence-reasons.html. Accessed 11/26/2004.

Badalian, L. et al. Neurological syndromes in Lyme disease in children, *Zh Nevropatol Psikhiatr Im S S Korsakova* 1994;94(3):3-6.

Bai, Y. et al. Spinal cord involvement in the nonhuman primate model of Lyme disease, *Lab Invest* 2004;84(2):160-72.

Barbour, Alan. *Lyme Disease:The Cause, the Cure, the Controversy*, Baltimore, MD:Johns Hopkins University Press, 1996.

Batalla, C. et al. Complete transitory atrioventricular block in Lyme disease, *Rev Esp Cardiol* 1999;52(7):529-31.

Bazovska, S. et al. Significance of specific antibody determination in Lyme borreliosis diagnosis, *Bratisl Lek Listy* 2001;102(10):454-7.

Beermann, C. et al. Lipoproteins from Borrelia burgdorferi applied in liposomes and presented by dendritic cells induce CD8(+) T-lymphocytes in vitro, *Cell Immunol* 2000;201(2):124-31.

Behan, W. and Stone, T. Enhanced neuronal damage by co-administration of quinolinic acid and free radicals, and protection by adenosine A2A receptor antagonists, *Br J Pharmacol* 2002;135(6):1435-42.

Behera, A. et al. Borrelia burgdorferi-induced expression of matrix metalloproteinases from human chondrocytes requires mitogen-activated protein kinase and janus kinase/signal transducer ad activator of transcription signaling pathways, *Infect Immun* 2004;72(5):2864-71.

————, et al. Induction of host matrix metalloproteinases by Borrelia burgdorferi differs in human and murine Lyme arthritis, *Infect Immun* 2005;73(1):126-34.

Beninger, R. et al. Picolinic acid blocks the neurotoxic but not the neuroexcitant properties of quinolinic acid in the rat brain: evidence from turning behavior and tyrosine hydroxylase immunohistochemistry, *Neuroscience* 1994;61(3):603-12.

Blaho, V. et al. Cyclooxygenase-2 modulates resolution but not severity of experimental Lyme arthritis. http://lifescienceweek. missouri.edu/uploads. abstract_pdf/vab712@1.pdf. Accessed 2/11/2005.

Blight, A. et al. Quinolinic acid accumulation and functional deficits following experimental spinal cord injury, *Brain* 1995;118(3):735-52.

Bock, Kenneth. Oxidative Modalities in Lyme Disease, audio tape, *8th International Bio-oxidative Conference*, May 16-18, 1997. www.treefarmtapes.com.

Boylan, J. Borrelia oxidative stress response regulator, BosR: a distinctive Zn-dependent transcriptional activator, *PNAS* 2003;100(20): 11684-9.

Bradley, J. et al. The persistence of spirochetal nucleic acids in active Lyme arthritis, *Ann Int Med* 1994;120(6):487-9.

Bransfield, P. et al. Evaluation of Antibiotic Treatment in Patients with Persistent Symptoms of Lyme Disease: An Ilads Position Paper. www.ilads.org/position2.html. Accessed 11/26/2004.

Brent, Hart. Treating Lyme disease with herbs and homeopathics in humans and their critters. www.healthcalls. net/hh_lyme.html. Accessed 5/20/2004.

Brisson, D. and Dykhuizen, D. OspC diversity in Borrelia burgdorferi: different hosts are different niches, *Genetics* 2004;168(2):713-22.

Brorson, O. and Brorson, S. In vitro conversion of Borrelia burgdorferi to cystic forms in spinal fluid, and transformation to mobile spirochetes by incubation in BSK-II medium, *Infection* 1998;26(3):144-50.

———. An in vitro study of the susceptibility of mobile and cystic forms of Borrelia burgdorferi to tinidazole, *Int Microbiol* 2004;7(2):139-42.

———. A rapid method for generating cystic forms of Borrelia burgdorferi, and their reversal to mobile spirochetes, *APMIS* 1998;106(12): 1131-4.

———. Transformation of cystic forms of Borrelia burgdorferi to normal, mobile spirochetes, *Infection* 1997;25(4):240-6.

Brown, C. and Reiner, S. Clearance of Borrelia burgdorferi may not be required for resistance to experimental Lyme arthritis, *Infect Immmun* 1998;66(5):2065-71.

Brown, E. et al. Modulation of immunity to Borrelia burgdorferi by ultraviolet radiation: differential effect on Th1 and Th2 immune responses, *Eur J Immunol* 1995;25(11):3017-22.

Bujak, D. et al. Clinical and neurocognitive features of the post Lyme syndrome, *J Rheumatol* 1996;23(8):1392-7.

Burgdorfer, Willy. The Complexity of Arthropod-borne Spirochetes (Borrelia spp.), Keynote Address, *12th International Conference on Lyme Disease and Other Spirochetal and Tick-borne Disorders*, April 9, 1999. www.canlyme.com/burgdorfer.html. Accessed 12.23.2004.

Burrascano, Joseph. Diagnostic Hints and Treatment Guidelines for Lyme and Other Tick Borne Illnesses, Fourteenth Edition, November 2002. www.ilads.org/burrascano_1102.html. Accessed 12/17/2004.

Cadavid, D. et al. Cardiac involvement in non-human primates infected with the Lyme disease spirochete Borrelia burgdorferi, *Lab Invest* 2004;84(11):1439-50.

Cadavid, D. et al. Isogenic serotypes of Borrelia turicatae show different localization in the brain and skin of mice, *Infect Immun* 2001;69(5): 3389-97.

Cadavid, D. et al. Localization of Borrelia burgdorferi in the nervous system and other organs in a nonhuman primate model of Lyme disease, *Lab Invest* 2000;80(7): 1043-54.

Cantorna, M. and Hayes, C. Vitamin A deficiency exacerbates murine Lyme arthritis, *J Infect Dis* 1996;174(4): 747-51.

Christopherson, J. et al. Destructive arthritis in vaccinated interferon gamma-deficient mice challenged with Borrelia burgdorferi: modulation by tumor necrosis factor alpha, *Clin and Diag Lab Immunol* 2003;10(1): 44-52.

Cluss, R. et al. Extracellular secretion of the Borrelia burgdorferi Oms28 porin and Bgp, a glycosaminoglycan binding protein, *Infect Immun* 2004;72(11):6279-86.

Cockhill, J. et al. Action of picolinic acid and structurally related puridine carboxylic acids on quinolinic acid-induced cortical cholinergic damage, *Brain Res* 1992;599(1):57-63.

Crawford, Amanda McQuade. The Herbal Treatment of Lyme Disease, Ojai, CA:Ojai Center of Phytotherapy, nd. xerox, 4 pages.

Dejmkova, H. et al. Seronegative Lyme arthritis caused by Borrelia garinii, *Clin Rheumatol* 2002;21(4):330-4.

Derdakova, M. et al. Interaction and transmission of two Borrelia burgdorferi sensu stricto strains in a tick-rodent maintenance system, *Appl Environ Microbiol* 2004;79(11):6783-8.

Dharmananda, Subhuti. Lyme Disease:Treatment with Chinese Herbs. www.itmonline.org/ arts/lyme.htm. Accessed 11/28/2004.

Diza, E. et al. Borrelia valaisiana in cerebrospinal fluid, *Emerg Infect Dis* 2004;10(9):1692-3.

Dotevall, L. et al. Astroglial and neuronal proteins in the cerebrospinal fluid as markers of CNS involvement in Lyme neuroborreliosis, *Eur J Neurol* 1999;6(2):169-78.

Drouin, E. et al. Molecular characterization of the OspA(161-175) T cell epitope associated with treatment-resistant Lyme arthritis differences among the three pathogenic species of Borrelia burgdorferi sensu lato, *J Autoimmun* 2004;23(3):281-92.

Dupeyron, A. et al. Sciatica, disk herniation, and neuroborreliosis. A report of four cases, *Joint Bone Spine* 2004;71(5):433-7.

Ebnet, K. et al. Borrelia burgdorferi activates NF-kB and is a potent inducer of chemokine and adhesion molecule gene expression in endothelial cells and fibroblasts, *Journal of Immunology* 1997;158:3285-3292.

Ekerfelt, C. et al. Asymptomatic Borrelia-seropositive individuals display the same incidence of Borrelia-specific interferon-gamma (IFN-gamma)-secreting cells in blood as patients with clinical Borrelia infection, *Clin Exp Immunol* 1999;115(3):498-502.

————. Compartmentalization of antigen specific cytokine responses to the central nervous system in CNS borreliosis: secretion of IFN-gamma predominates over IL-4 secretion in response to outer surface proteins of Lyme disease Borrelia spirochetes, *J Neuroimmunol* 1997;79(2):155-62.

Eiffert, H. et al. Acute peripheral facial palsy in Lyme disease—a distal neuritis at the infection site, *Neuropediatrics* 2004;35(5):267-73.

————. Nondifferentiation between Lyme disease spirochetes from vector ticks and human cerebrospinal fluid, *J Infec Dis* 1995;171(2):476-0.

Fallon, Brian. Heavy Metal: Matrix Metalloproteinases in Lyme Disease. Medscape. www.medscape.com/viewarticle/412985. Accessed 12/24/2005.

———— and Nields, J. Lyme disease: a neuropsychiatric illness, *Am J Psychiatry* 1994;151(11):1571-83.

Fang Ting Liang and Philip, Mario. Analysis of antibody response to invariable regions of VlsE, the variable surface antigen of Borrelia burgdorferi, *Infection and Immunity* 1999;67(12):6702-6.

Fivaz, B. and Petney, T. Lyme disease—a new disease in southern Africa? *J S Afr Vet Assoc* 1989;60(3):155-8.

Garcia, R. et al. Elastase is the human neutrophil granule protein responsible for the in vitro killing of the Lyme disease spirochete Borrelia burgdorferi, *Infection and Immunity* 1998;66(4):1408-12.

Gasse, T. et al. Neopterin production and tryptophan degradation in acute Lyme neuroborreliosis verses late Lyme encephalopathy, *Eur J Clin Chem Clin Biochem* 1994;32(9):685-9.

Gebbia, J. et al. Borrelia spirochetes upregulate release and activation of matrix metalloproteinase gelatinase B (MMP-9) and collagenase 1 (MMP-1) in human cells, *Infect Immun* 2001;69(1):456-62.

Georgilis, K. et al. Fibroblasts protect the Lyme disease spirochete, Borrelia burgdorferi, from ceftriaxone in vitro, *J Infect Dis* 1992;166(2):440-4.

Ginsberg, Howard. *Ecology and Environmental Management of Lyme Disease*, New Brunswick, NJ: Rutgers University Press, 1993.

Girschick, H. et al. Intracellular persistence of Borrelia burgdorferi in human synovial cells, *Rheumatol Int* 1996;16(3):125-32.

Goldberg, Burton and Trivieri, Larry. *Chronic fatigue, Fibromyalgia and Lyme Disease*, Second Edition, Berkeley, CA:Celestial Arts, 2004.

Goldhagen, H. and Rawlings, J. Clinical Aspects of Lyme Disease: Dermatologic, Cardiac, GI, and Gestational. Medscape. www.medscape.com/viewarticle/4184 40. Accessed 10/23/2004.

————. Fighting back: how B. burgdorferi persists. Medscape. www.medscape.com/viewarticle.4184 48. Accessed 10/23/2004.

————. Lyme Disease Controversies. Medscape. www.medscape.com/viewarticle/418442. Accessed 2/1/2005.

Goldings, Audrey. Controversies in Neuroborreliosis. www.ilads.org/goldings.html. Accessed 12/19/2004.

Goss, Matthew. Lyme Disease Research and Perspective. 20 pages. www.matthewgoss.org. Accessed 11/3/04.

Gray, J.S. et al, editors. *Lyme Borreliosis: Biology, Epidemiology, and Control*, NY:CABI Publishing, 2002.

Greenberg, H. et al. Sleep quality in Lyme disease, *Sleep* 1995;18(10):912-6.

Gruber, Joachim. Long-term Inflammation in Lyme Borreliosis: A Medline-literature Survey, February 3, 1999. www.lymenet.de/literatur/niches.htm. Accessed 12/19/2004.

Gruntar, I. et al. Conversion of Borrelia garinii cystic forms to motile spirochetes in vivo, *APMIS* 2001;109(5):383-8.

Grygorczuk, S. et al. Serum and cerebrospinal fluid concentration of inflammatory proteins MIP-1-alpha and MIP-1-beta and of interleukin 8 in the course of borreliosis, *J Neurochir Pol* 2003; 37(1):73-87.

Guardigli, M. et al. Evaluation of reactive oxygen species production in Kupffer cells by chemiluminescence, *12th International Symposium on Bioluminescence and Chemiluminescence*, www.lumiweb.com/sym2002/abstracts. Accessed 12/29/2004.

Guerau-de-Arellano, M. and Huber, B. Development of autoimmunity in Lyme arthritis, *Curr Opin Rheumatol* 2002;14(4):388-93.

Halouzka, J. et al. Isolation of Borrelia afzelii from overwintering Culex pipiens biotype molestus mosquitoes, *Infection* 1999;27(4):275-7.

Halperin, J. Central nervous system Lyme disease, *Curr Infect Dis Rep* 2004;6(4):298-304.

————. Neuroborreliosis: central nervous system involvement, *Semin Neurol* 1997;17(1):19-24.

———— and Golightly, M. Lyme borreliosis in Bell's palsy. Long Island neuroborreliosis collaborative study group, *Neurology* 1992;42(7):1268-70.

———— and Heyes, M. Neuroactive kynurenines in Lyme borreliosis *Neurology* 1992;42(1):43-50.

Hannier, S. et al. Characterization of the B-cell inhibitory protein factor in Ixodes ricinus tick saliva: a potential role in enhanced Borrelia burgdorferi transmission, *Immunology* 2004;113(3):401-8.

Harvey, W. and Salvato, P. "Lyme Disease": ancient engine of an unrecognized borreliosis pandemic? *Medical Hypothesis* 2003;60(5):742-59.

He, S. et al. Review on acupuncture treatment of peripheral facial paralysis during the past decade, *J Tradit Chin Med* 1995;15(1):63-7.

Helbing-Sheafe, Hannelore. *Lyme Disease:Alternative Medicine Can Help*, Olympia, WA:Huckleberry Hill Press, 2003.

Henneberg, J. and Neubert, U. Borrelia burgdorferi group: in vitro antibiotic sensitivity, *Orv Hetil* 2002;143(21):1195-8.

Hernandez-Novoa, B. et al. Utility of a commercial immunoblot kit (BAG-Borreila blot) in the diagnosis of the preliminary stages of Lyme disease, *Diagn Microbiol Infect Dis* 2003;47(1):321-9.

Heron, P. and Daya, S. 17Beta-estradiol attenuates quinolinic acid insult in the rat hippocampus, *Metab Brain Dis* 2001;16(3-4):187-98.

Herzer, P. et al. Lyme arthritis: clinical features, serological, and radiographic findings of cases in Germany, *Kim Wochenschr* 1986;64(5):206-15.

Heyes, M. et al. Elevated cerebrospinal fluid quinolinic acid levels are associated with region-specific cerebral volume loss in HIV infection, *Brain* 2001;124(5):1033-42.

———. Human microglia convert L-tryptophan into neurotoxin quinolinic acid, *Biochem J* 1996;320:595-7.

———. Sources of the neurotoxin quinolinic acid in the brain of HIV-1 infected patients and retrovirus-infected macaques, *The FASEB Journal*, 1998;12:881-96.

Hoffman, Ronald. *Lyme Disease*, New Canaan, CT:Keats, 1994.

Holub, M. et al. Lymphocyte subset numbers in cerebrospinal fluid: comparisons of tick-borne encephalitis and neuroborreliosis, *Acta Neurol Scand* 2002;106(5):302-8.

Hu, L. et al. Host metalloproteinases in Lyme arthritis, *Arthritis Rheum* 2001;44(6):1401-10.

Hubalek, Z. and Halouzka, J. Distribution of Borrelia burgdorferi sensu lato genomic groups in Europe, a review, *Eur J Epidemiol* 1997;13(8):951-7.

Hubalek, Z. et al. Investigation of haematophagous arthropods for borreliae-summarized data, 1988-1996, *Folia Parasitol (Praha)* 1998;45(1):67-72.

Hulinska, Dagmar. Influence of zinc on Borrelia garinii, *VII International Congress on Lyme Borreliosis*, abstracts, San Francisco, CA:J.D.Gubler, 1996, 323.

Hunt, L. Ocular Lyme disease, *Insight* 1996;21(2):56-7.

Huppertz, H. et al. Ocular manifestations in children and adolescents with Lyme arthritis, *Br J Ophthalmol* 1999;83(10):1149-52.

Ilads. ILADS' Position Paper on the CDC's Statement Regarding Lyme Diagnosis. www.ilads.org/cdc_paper.html. Accessed 11/26/2004.

Infante-Duarte, C. and Kamradt, T. Lipopeptides of Borrelia burgdorferi outer surface proteins induce Th1 phenotype development in alphabeta T-cell receptor transgenic mice, *Infect Immun* 1997;65(10):4094-99.

Isogai, E. et al. Cytokines in the serum and brain in mice infected with distinct species of Lyme disease borrelia, *Microb Pathog* 1996;21(6):413-9.

Jacobsen, M. et al. Clonal accumulation of activated CD8+ T cells in the central nervous system during the early phase of neuroborreliosis, *J Infect Dis* 2003;187(6):963-73.

Jalaudin, M. Methylcobalmin treatment of Bell's palsy, *Methods Find Exp Clin Pharmacol* 1995;17:539-44.

Jernigan, David. *Surviving Lyme Disease Using Alternative Medicine*, Wichita, KS:Seomerleyton Press, 1999.

Jhamandas, K. et al. The 1993 Upjohn Award Lecture. Quinolinic acid induced brain neurotransmitter deficits: modulation b endogenous excitoxin antagonists, *Can J Physiol Pharmacol* 1994;72(12):1473-82.

Johnson, L. and Stricker, R. Treatment of Lyme disease:a medicological assessment, *Expert Rev Anti Infect Ther* 2004;2(4):533-57.

Johnson, Lorraine. Lyme Disease; Two Standards of Care. www.ilads.org/insurance.html. Accessed 11/26/2004.

Johnson, Russell, editor. *The Biology of Parasitic Spirochetes*, NY:Academic Press, 1976.

Kaiser, R. Clinical courses of acute and chronic neuroborreliosis following treatment with ceftriaxone, *Nervenarzt* 2004;75(6):553-7.

Kaplan, Richard, editor. Neuro-psychological Aspects of Lyme Disease, *Applied Neuropsychology*, Special Issue, 1999;6(1):entire publication.

Karlan, Arno. *Biography of a Germ*, NY:Random House, 2000.

Kazragis, R. et al. In vivo activities of ceftriaxone and vancomycin against Borrelia spp. in the mouse brain and other sites, *Antimicrob Agents Chemother* 1996;40(11):2632-6.

Keane-Meyers, A. and Nickell, S. T cell subset-dependent modulation of immunity to Borrelia burgdorferi in mice, *J Immunol* 1995;154(4):1770-6.

Kenefick, K. et al. Borrelia burgdorferi stimulates release of interleukin-1 activity from bovine peripheral blood monocytes, *Infect Immun* 1992;60(9):3630-4.

Kida, E. and Matyja, E. Prevention of quinolinic acid neurotoxicity in rat hippocampus in vitro by zinc. Ultrastructural observations, *Neuroscience* 1990;37(2):347-52.

Kinderlehrer, Daniel. Healing Lyme Disease: An Integrated Approach to Curing. www.lymesite.com. Accessed 5/29/04.

Kirchner, A. et al. Upregulation of matrix metalloproteinase-9 in the cerebrospinal fluid of patients with acute Lyme neuroborreliosis, *J Neurol Neurosurg Psychiatry* 2000;68(3): 368-71.

Klempner, M. et al. Invasion of human skin fibroblasts by the Lyme disease spirochete, Borrelia burgdorferi, *J Infect Dis* 1993;167(5):1074-81.

———. Two controlled trials of antibiotic treatment in patients with persistent symptoms and a history of Lyme disease, *N Eng J Med* 2001;345(2):85-92.

Klinghardt, Dietrich. The Use of Pharmax Neutriceuticals in the Treatment of Chronic Lyme Disease, *Explore* 2002;11(4):no page numbers available (6 pages).

Krause, Richard, editor. *Emerging Infections*, NY:Academic press, 1998.

Kosik-Bogacka, D. Detection of Borrelia burgdorferi sensu lato in mosquitoes (Culicidae) in recreational areas of the city of Szczecin, *Ann Agri Environ Med* 2002;9(1):55-7.

———— et al. The prevalence of spirochete Borrelia burgdorferi sensu lato in ticks Ixodes ricinus and mosquitoes Aedes spp. within a selected recreational area in the city of Szezecin, *Ann Agric Environ Med* 2004;11(4):105-8.

Lane, R. et al. Anti-arthropod saliva antibodies among residents of a community at high risk for Lyme disease in California, *Am J Trop Med Hyg* 1999;61(5):850-9.

———— et al. Risk factors for Lyme disease in a small rural community in northern California, *Am J Epidemiol* 1992;136(11):1358-68.

Lang, Denise. *Coping With Lyme Disease*, Third Edition, NY:Henry Holt, 2004.

Lange, R. and Seyyedi, S. Evidence of a Lyme borreliosis infection from the viewpoint of laboratory medicine, *Int J Med Microbiol* 2002;291(Suppl 33):120-4.

Latov, N. et al. Neuropathy and cognitive impairment following vaccination with the OspA protein of Borrelia burgdorferi, *J Peripher Nerv Syst* 2004 Sep;9(3):165-7.

Lederberg, Joshua, et al, editors. *Emerging Infections:Microbial Threats to Health in the United States*, Washington, D.C.:National Academy Press, 1992.

Leong, J. et al. Different classes of proteoglycans contribute to the attachment of Borrelia burgdorferi in cultured endothelial and brain cells, *Infect Immun* 1998;66(3):994-9.

Li, Y. et al. Efficacy of acupuncture and moxibustion in treating Bell's palsy: a multicenter randomized controlled trial in China, *Chin Med J (Engl)* 2004;117(10):1502-6.

Liang, F. et al. Borrelia burgdorferi changes its surface antigenic expression in response to host immune responses, *Infect Immun* 2004;72(10):5759-67.

————. An immune evasion mechanism for spirochetal persistence in Lyme borreliosis, *J Exp Med* 2002;195(4):415-22.

————. Protective niche for Borrelia burgdorferi to evade humoral immunity, *Am J Pathol* 2004;165(3):977-85.

Limbach, F. et al. Treatment resistant Lyme arthritis caused by Borrelia garinii, *Am Rheum Dis* 2001;60(3):284-6.

Logigian, E. et al. Reversible cerebral hypoperfusion in Lyme encephalopathy, *Neurology* 1997;49(6):1661-70.

Lomholt, H. et al. Long-term serological follow-up of patients treated for chronic cutaneous borreliosis or culture-positive erythema migrans, *Acta Derm Venereol* 2000;80(5):362-6.

Luger, S. Lyme disease transmitted by a biting fly, *New England Journal of Medicine* 1990;322(24):1752.

Magnarelli, L. et al. The etiologic agent of Lyme disease in deer flies, horse flies, and mosquitoes, *J Infect Dis* 1986;154(2):355-8.

Miklossy, J. et al. Borrelia burgdorferi persists in the brain in chronic Lyme neuroborreliosis and may be associated with Alzheimer's disease, *Journal of Alzheimer's Disease* 2004;6(6):no page numbers available.

Miller, J. and Stevenson, B. Increased expression of Borrelia burgdorferi factor H-binding surface proteins during transmission from ticks to mice, *Int J Med Microbiol* 2004;293(Suppl 37):120-5.

Miller, L. et al. Live Borrelia burgdorferi preferentially activate interleukin-1 beta gene expression and protein synthesis over the interleukin=1 receptor antagonist, *J Clin Invest* 1992;90(3):906-12.

Miller, Lloyd, Notes from the Ninth Lyme Disease Foundation Annual Scientific Conference, *Lymenet Newsletter* 1996;4(10): no page numbers available.

Mitra, M. and Nandi, A. Cyanocobalmin in chronic Bell's palsy, *Ind Med Assoc* 1959;33:129-31.

Montgomery, R. and Malawista, S. Borrelia burgdorferi and the macrophage: routine annihilation but occasional haven? *Parisitol Today* 1994;10(4):154-7.

Montgomery, R. et al. The fate of Borrelia burgdorferi, the agent for Lyme disease, in mouse macrophages. Destruction, survival, recovery. *J Immunol* 1993;150(3):909-15.

Murgia, R. et al. Cystic forms of Borrelia burgdorferi sensu lato: induction, development, and the role of RpoS, *Wien Klin Wochenschr* 2002; 114(13-14):574-9.

———— and Cinco, M. Induction of cystic forms by different stress conditions in Borrelia burgdorferi, *APMIS* 2004;112(1):57-62.

Mursic, V. et al. Formation and cultivation of Borrelia burgdorferi spheroplast L-form variants, *Infection* 1996;24(3):218-26.

Nanagara, R. et al. Ultrastructural demonstration of spirochetal antigens in synovial fluid and synovial membrane in chronic Lyme disease: possible factors contributing to persistence of organisms, *Hum Pathol* 1996;27(10):1025-34.

Narasimban, S. et al. Borrelia burgdorferi transcriptome in the central nervous system of non-human primates, *Proc Natl Acad Sci USA* 2003;100(26):15953-8.

Nardelli, D. et al. Association of CD4+ CD25+ T cells with prevention of severe destructive arthritis in Borrelia burgdorferi-vaccinated and challenged gamma interferon-deficient mice treated with anti-interleukin 17 antibody, *Clin Diag Lab Immunol* 2004;11(6):1075-84.

Nicolson, G. et al. Diagnosis and integrative treatment of intracellular bacterial infections in chronic fatigue and fibromyalgia syndromes, Gulf War illness, rheumatoid arthritis and other chronic disorders, *Clinical Practice of Alternative Medicine* 2000;1(2):42-102.

Oksi, J. et al. Borrelia burgdorferi detected by culture and PCR in clinical relapse of disseminated Lyme borreliosis, *Ann Med* 1999;31(3): 225-32.

————. Inflammatory brain changes in
Lyme borreliosis. A report on three
patients and a review of literature,
Brain 1996;119(Pt 6):2143-54.

Pachner, A. et al. Central and peripheral
nervous system infection, immunity,
and inflammation in the NHP model
of Lyme borreliosis, *Ann Neurol*
2001;50(3):330-8.

————. Genotype determines phenotype in experimental Lyme
borreliosis, *Ann Neurol* 2004;56(30):
361-70.

————. Interleukin-6 is expressed at
high levels in the CNS in Lyme
neuroborreliosis, *Neurology*
1997;49(1):147-52.

Pal, U. et al. TROSPA, an Ixodes
scapularis receptor for Borrelia
burgdorferi, *Cell* 2004;119(4):457-68.

Parveen, N. and Leong, J. Identification
of a candidate glycosaminoglycan-
binding adhesin of the Lyme disease
spirochete Borrelia burgdorferi, *Mol
Microbiol* 2000;35(5):1220-34.

Patarca-Montero, R. et al. Immuno-
therapy of chronic fatigue syndrome:
therapeutic interventions aimed at
modulating the Th1/Th2 cytokine
expression balance, *Journal of Chronic
Fatigue Syndrome* 2001;8(1):12-23.

Pavis, Charles. Overview of the
pathogenic spirochetes, *Journal of
Spirochetal and Tick-borne Illnesses*
1994;1(1):no page numbers available.

Pechova, J. et al. Tick salivary gland
extract-activated transmission of
Borrelia afzelii spirochetes, *Folia
Parasitologica* 2002;49:153-9.

Peltomaa, Mikka. Lyme Borreliosis in
Neurootological Patients and the
Prevalence of Borrelia burgdorferi
S.L. in urban Ixodes ricinus ticks,
Helsinki, 1999, Academic
Dissertation.

Perides, G. et al. Matrix Metalloproteinases in the cerebrospinal fluid of
patients with Lyme neuroborreliosis, *J
Infect Dis* 1998;177(2):401-8.

Peters, S. et al. Zinc selectively blocks the
action of N-methyl-aspartate on
cortical neurons, *Science* 1987;
236(4801):589-93.

Phillips, S. et al. A proposal for the
reliable culture of Borrelia
burgdorferi from patients with
chronic Lyme disease, even from
those previously aggressively treated,
Infection 1998;26(6):364-7.

Picken, M. et al. A two-year prospective
study to compare culture and
polymerase chain reaction amplification for the detection and
diagnosis of Lyme borreliosis, *Mol
Pathol* 1997;50(4):186-93.

Potter, M. et al. Role of osteopontin in
murine Lyme arthritis and host
defense against Borrelia burgdorferi,
Infect Immun 2002;79(3):1372-81.

Priem, S. Detection of Borrelia
burgdorferi by polymerase chain
reaction in synovial membrane, but
not in synovial fluid from patients
with persisting Lyme arthritis after
antibiotic therapy, *Ann Rheum Dis*
1998;57(2):118-21.

Program and abstracts of the 14th
International Scientific Conference on
Lyme Disease and Other Tick-borne
Disorders, April 21.23, 2001,
Hartford, CT.

Qin, Z. et al. Nuclear factor-kappa B contributes to excitotoxin-induced apoptosis in rat striatum, *Mol Pharmacol* 1998;53(1):33-42.

Qiu, W. et al. Genetic exchange and plasmid transfers in Borrelia burgdorferi sensu stricto revealed by three-way genome comparisons and multilocus sequence typing, *Proc Natl Acad Sci USA* 2004; 101(39):14150-5.

Rasley, A. et al. Borrelia burgdorferi induces inflammatory mediator production by murine microglia, *J Neuroimmunol* 2002;130(1-2):22-31.

Richter, D. et al. Relationship of a novel Lyme disease spirochete, Borrelia spielmani sp. nov., with its hosts in central Europe, *Appl Environ Microbiol* 2004;70(11):6414-9.

Riviere, G. et al. Molecular and immunological evidence of oral Treponema in human brain and their association with Alzheimer's disease, *Oral Microbiol Immunol* 2002;17(2):113-8.

Rock, B. et al. Role of microglia in central nervous system infections, *Clinical Microbiology Reviews* 2004;17(4):942-64.

Rubel, Joanne. Spirochetal Cysts, L-forms, and Blebs: Observations from 1905 to 2002. 48 pages, 142 abstracts. www.lymeinfo.net/medical/LDBibliography.pdf. Accessed 2.11.2005.

Saier, Milton and Garcia-Lara, Jorge, editors. *The Spirochetes: Molecular and Cellular Biology*, Norfolk, England: Horizon Scientific press, 2001.

Salazar, J. et al. Coevolution of markers of innate and adaptive immunity in skin and peripheral blood of patients with erythema migrans, *J Immunol* 2003;171(5):2660-70.

Santamaria, A. et al. Copper blocks quinolinic acid neurotoxicity in rats: contribution of antioxidant systems, *Free Rad Biol Med* 2003;35(4):418-27.

Santamaria, J. et al. Protective effects of the antioxidant selenium on quinolinic acid-induced neurotoxicity in rats: in vitro and in vivo studies, *J Neurochem* 2003;86(2):479-88.

Schardt, F. Clinical effects of fluconazole in patients with neuroborreliosis, *Eur J Med Res* 2004;9(7):334-6.

Schell, R. et al. Anti-IL-17 therapy halts arthritis in mice with Lyme disease, *Infect Immun* 2003;71:3437-3442.

Schutzer, Steven. *Lyme Disease:Molecular and Immunological Approaches*, Plainview, NY:Cold Spring Harbor Laboratory Press, 1992.

Schutzer, S. et al. Simultaneous expression of Borrelia OspA and OspC and IgM response in cerebrospinal fluid in early neurologic Lyme disease, *J Clin Invest* 1997;100(4): 763-7.

Seifert, E. et al. Neurogenic inflammation and area of involvement of the facial nerve of the rat, *Laryngorhino-otologie* 1994;73(6):342-5.

Seshu, J. et al. Dissolved oxygen levels alter gene expression and antigen profiles in Borrelia burgdorferi, *Infect Immun* 2004;72(3):1580-6.

Shanafelt, M. et al. Modulation of murine Lyme borreliosis by interruption of the B7/CD28 T-cell costimulatory pathway, *Infect Immun* 1998;66(1):266-71.

Sherr, Virginia. Two Detailed Case Histories Involving Patients with Coinfections—Babesia, Ehrlichiosis, and Lyme Disease. www.ilads.org/sherr4.html. Accessed 11/26/2004.

Silverstein, Alvin, et al. *Lyme Disease: The Great Imitator*, Lebanon, NJ:Avstar Publishing, 1990.

Stanek, G. Epidemiology of borrelia infections in Austria, *Zentralbl Bakteriol Mikrobiol* 1987;263(3):442-9.

———. Erythema migrans and serodiagnosis by enzyme immunoassay and immunoblot with three borrelia species, *Wien Klin Wochenschr* 1999;111(22-23):951-6.

Steere, A. et al. Autoimmune mechanisms in antibiotic treatment-resistant Lyme arthritis, *J Autoimmun* 2001;16(3):263-8.

———. Binding of outer surface protein A and human lymphocyte function-associated antigen 1 peptides to HLA-DR molecules associated with antibiotic treatment-resistant Lyme arthritis, *Arthritis Rheum* 2003;48(2):534-40.

——— and Glickstein, L. Elucidation of Lyme arthritis, *Immunology*, 2004;4: 143-152.

Straubinger, Reinhard. PCR-based quantification of Borrelia burgdorferi organisms in canine tissues over a 500-day postinfection period, *Ann Clin Microbiol* 2000;38(6):2191-99.

Stricker, R.B. and Lautin, A. The Lyme Wars:time to listen, *Expert Opin Investig Drugs* 2003 Oct;12(10): 1069-14.

Stricker, R. and Winger, E. Decreased CD57 lymphocyte subset in patients with chronic Lyme disease, *Immunol Lett* 2001;76(1):43-8.

Strle, F. Treatment of borrelial lymphocytoma, *Infection* 1996;24(1):80-4.

——— et al. Solitary borrelial lymphocytoma: a report of 36 cases, *Infection* 1992;20(4):201-6.

Tarasow, E. et al. Neuroborreliosis: CT and MRI findings in 14 cases. Preliminary communications, *J Neurol Neurochir Pol* 2001;35(5):803-13.

Tokarz, R. et al. Combined effects of blood and temperature shift on Borrelia burgdorferi gene expression as determined by whole genome DNA assay, *Infect Immun* 2004;72(9): 5419-32.

Treib, J. et al. Chronic fatigue syndrome in patients with Lyme borreliosis, *Eur Neurol* 2000;43(2):107-9.

Valesova, H. et al. Long-term results in patients with Lyme arthritis following treatment with ceftriaxone, *Infection* 1996;24(1):98-102.

Vasilu, V. et al. Heterogeneity of Borrelia burgdorferi sensu lato demonstrated by an OspA-type-specific PCR in synovial fluid from patients with Lyme arthritis, *Med Microbiol Immunol* 1998;187(2):97-102.

Vijay, S. et al. Diagnosis of Lyme borreliosis by a whole-blood gamma interferon assay for cell-mediated immune responses, *Clin Diag Lab Immun* 1999;6(3):445.

Vredevoe, L. et al. Detection and characterization of Borrelia bissettii in rodents from the central California coast, *J Med Entomol* 2004;41(4): 736-45.

Walker, Lynne. Lyme Disease: More Common Than You Realize, audio tape, *17th Annual AANP Convention*, August 14-17, 2002. www.treefarmtapes.com.

Wang, G. et al. Evidence for frequent OspC gene transfer between Borrelia valaisiana sp. nov. and other Lyme disease spirochetes, *FEMS Microbiol Lett* 1999;177(2):289-96.

Wang. W. et al. Lyme neuroborreliosis:evidence for persistent up-regulation of Borrelia burgdorferi-reactive cells secreting interferon-gamma, *Scand J Immunol* 1995;42(6):694-700.

Weger, W. and Mullegger, R. Histopathology and immunohistochemistry of dermatoborreliosis, *Acta Dermatovenerologica* 2001;10(4):no page numbers available.

Widhe, M. et al. Borrelia-specific interferon-gamma and interleukin-4 secretion in cerebrospinal fluid and blood during Lyme borreliosis in humans: associations and clinical outcomes, *J Infect Dis* 2004;189-200.

Winston, David. Botanical Treatment for Today's Infectious Diseases. Audio tape. *Southwest Conference on Botanical Medicine*, 2000.

————. Experimental Herbal Protocols. Audio tape. *Medicines From the Earth Conference*, 1999.

————. Experimental Protocols for Lyme Disease, 2004, self-published, 5 pages.

Yagi, N. et al. The effect of steroid and CH3 vitamin B-12 on peripheral facial paralysis, *Otologia Fukuoaka* 1981;74:1613.

Yamane, K. et al. Clinical efficacy of intravenous plus oral mecobalmin in patients with peripheral neuropathy using vibration perception thresholds as an indicator or improvement, *Curr Ther Res* 1995;56:656-70.

Yanagihara, N. et al. Edematous swelling of the facial nerve in Bell's palsy, *Acta Otolaryngol* 2000;120(5):667-71.

Yilmaz, M. et al. Serum cytokine levels in Bell's palsy, *J Neurol Sci* 2002;197(1-2):69-72.

Yushchenko, M. et al. Matrix metalloproteinase-9 (MMP-9) in human cerebrospinal fluid (CSF): elevated levels are primarily related to CSF cell count, *J Neuroimmunol* 2000;110(1-2):244-51.

Zajkowaska, J. et al. Analysis of some peripheral blood lymphocyte subsets in relation to Borrelia burgdorferi antibodies in patients with Lyme disease, *Rocz Akad Med Bialymst* 2000;45:184-98.

————. Neurologic syndromes in Lyme disease, *Pol Merkuriusz Lek* 2000;9(50):584-8.

Zakovska, A. et al. Positive findings of Borrelia burgdorferi in Culex (Culex) pipiens pipiens larvae in the surrounding of Brno city determined by the PCR method, *Ann Agric Environ Med* 2002;9(2):257-9.

Zambrano, M. et al. Borreila burgdorferi binds to, invades, and colonizes native Type I collagen lattices, *Infect Immun* 2004;72(6):3138-46.

Zhang, J. 80 cases of peripheral facial paralysis treated by acupuncture with vibrating shallow insertion, *J Tradit Chin Med* 1999;19:44-7.

Zhang, Qingcai. Treating Lyme Disease with Modern Chinese Medicine. 13 pages. www.dr-zhang.com. Accessed 5/28/04.

BABESIA:

Adelson, M. et al. Prevalence of borrelia burgdorferi, Bartonella spp., Babesia microti, and Anaplasma phagocytophila in Ixodes scapularis ticks collected in Northern New Jersey, *J Clin Microbiol* 2004;42(6):2799-801.

Belongia, E. Epidemiology and impact of coinfections acquired from Ixodes ticks, *Vector Borne Zoonotic Dis* 2002;2(4):265-73.

Cunha, Burke. Babesiosis. Emedicine, www.emedicine.com. Accessed 2/1/2005.

Henderson, Sean. Babesiosis. Emedicine, www.emedicine.com. Accessed 12/12/2004.

Herwaldt, B. et al. Endemic babesiosis in another eastern state: New jersey, *Emerging Infectious Diseases* 2003;9(2), no page numbers available.

Krause, P. et al. Concurrent Lyme disease and babesiosis: evidence for increased severity and duration of illness, *JAMA* 1996; 275(21):1657-60.

Mitchell, P. et al. Immunoserologic evidence of coinfection with Borrelia burgdorferi, Babesia microti, and human granulocytic Ehrlichia species in residents of Wisconsin and Minnesota, *J Clin Microbiol* 1996;34(3):724-7.

Moro, M. et al. Increased arthritis severity in mice coinfected with Borrelia burgdorferi and Babesia microti, *J Infect Dis* 2002; 186(3): 428-31.

Nagai, A. et al. Growth-inhibitory effects of artesunate, pyrimethamine, and pamaquine against Babesia equi and babesia caballi in in vitro cultures, *Antimicrobial Agents and Chemotherapy* 2003;47(2):800-803.

Oleson, C. et al. Transverse myelitis secondary to coexistent Lyme disease and babesiosis, *J Spinal Cord Med* 2003;26(2):168-71.

Skotarczak, B. et al. Molecular evidence of coinfection of Borrelia burgdorferi sensu lato, human granulocytic ehrlichiosis agent, and Babesia microti in ticks from northwestern Poland, *J Parasitol* 2003;89(1):194-6.

Steere, A. et al. Prospective study of coinfection in patients with erythema migrans, *Clin Infect Dis* 2003;36(8):1078-81.

BARTONELLA:

Binggeli, S. et al. Molecular and cellular basis of bacterial persistence in the infected host. www.biozentrum. unibas.ch/report. Accessed 11/6/12004.

Breitschwerdt, E. and Kordick, Dorsey. Bartonella infection in animals: carriership, reservoir potential, pathogenicity, and zoonotic potential for human infection, *Clinical Microbiology Reviews* 2000;13(3):428-38.

Bruckert, F. et al. Sternal abscess due to Bartonella (Rochalimaea) henselae in a renal transplant patient, *Skeletal Radiol* 1997; 26(7):431-3.

Burgess, A. and Anderson, B. Outer membrane proteins of Bartonella henselae and their interaction with human endothelial cells, *Microbial Pathogenesis* 1998;25(3):157-64.

Chang, C. et al. Molecular evidence of bartonella spp. in questing adult Ixodes pacificus ticks in California, *J Clin Microbiol* 2001;39(4):1221-6.

Chung, Crystal, et al. Bartonella spp. DNA associated with biting flies from California, *Emerg Infect Dis* 2004;10(7):no page numbers avail.

Dehio, C. Biozentrum Biennial Report 2002-2003. www.biozentrum.unibas. ch. Accessed 12/15/2004.

————. Molecular and cellular basis of bartonella pathogenesis, *Annu Rev Microbiol* 2004;58:365-90.

———— et al. Interaction of Bartonella henselae with endothelial cells results in bacterial aggregation on cell surface and the subsequent engulf-ment and internalization of the bacterial aggregate by a unique structure, the invasome, *Journal of Cell Science* 1997;110(18):2141-54.

Edwards, Brian. Bartonella. Emedicine. www.emedicine.com. Accessed 2/1/2005.

Eskow, E. et al. Concurrent infection of the central nervous system by Borrelia burgdorferi and Bartonella henselae: evidence for a novel tick-borne disease complex, *Arch Neurol* 2001;58(9):1357-63.

Fuhrmann, Oliver, et al. Bartonella henselae induces NF-kB-dependent upregulation of adhesion molecules in cultured human endothelial cells:possible role of outer membrane proteins as pathogenic factors, *Infection and Immunity* 2001;69(8): 5088-97.

Hofmeister, E. et al. Cosegregation of a novel Bartonella species with Borrelia burgdorferi and Babesia microti in Peromyscus leucopus, *J Infect Dis* 1998;177(2):409-16.

Minnick, M. et al. cell entry and the pathogenesis of bartonella infections, *Trends Microbiol* 1996;4(9):343-7.

Musso, D. et al. Lack of bactericidal effect of antibiotics except aminoglycosides on Bartonella (Rochalimaea) henselae, *Journal of Antimicrobial Chemotherapy* 1995;36:101-8.

Musso, T. et al. Interaction of Bartonella henselae with the murine macrophage cell line J774: Infection and proinflammatory response, *Infection and Immunity* 2001;69(10):5974-80.

Numazaki, Kei. Bartonella henselae and Coxiella burnetii infection and the karasaki disease, *J Appl Sci Environ Mgt* 2004;8(1):11-12.

Pappalardo, Brandee, et al. Immunopathology of Bartonella vinsonii (berkhoffii) in experimentally infected dogs, *Veterinary Immunology and Immuno-pathology* 2001;83(3-4):125-47.

Podsiadly E. et al. Bartonella henselae and Borrelia burgdorferi infections of the central nervous system, *Ann N Y Acad Sci* 2003;990:404-6.

Resto-Ruiz, S. et al. The role of the host immune response in pathogenesis of Bartonella henselae, *DNA Cell Biol* 2003;22(6):431-40.

Rolain, Jean-Marc, et al. Culture and antibiotic susceptibility of Bartonella quintana in human erythrocytes, *Am Soc Micro Antimicro Agents Chemother* 2003;47(2):614-9.

Schmid, Michael, et al. The VirB type IV secretion system of Bartonella henselae mediates invasion, proinflammatory activation and antiapoptic protection of endothelial cells, *Molecular Microbiology* 2004;52(1):81.

Schmidt, A., editor. *Bartonella and Afipia Species, Emphasizing Bartonella henselae*, Basel, Switzerland:Karger, 1998.

Schmiederer, Michael, et al. Intracellular induction o the Bartonella henselae virB operon by human endothelial cells, *Infection and Immunity* 2001;69(10):6495-6502.

Schulein, Ralf, et al. Invasion and persistent intracellular colonization of erythrocytes: A unique parasitic strategy of the emerging pathogen Bartonella, *Journal of Experimental Medicine* 2001;193(9):1077-86.

Tappero, Jordan, et al. Bacillary angiomatosis and bacillary splenitis in immunocompetent adults, *Ann Intern Med* 1993;118(5):363-5.

Windsor, J.J. Cat-scratch disease: epidemiology, aetiology, and treatment, *Br J Biomed Sci* 2001;58(2):101-10.

EHRLICHIA:

Abuhammour, Walid. Ehrlichiosis. Emedicine. www.emedicine.com. Accessed 2/1/2005.

Belongia, E.A. et al. Clinical and epidemiological features of early Lyme disease and human granulocytic ehrlichiosis in Wisconsin, *Clin Infect Dis* 1999;29(6):1472-7.

Cao, W.C. et al. Prevalence of Anaplasma phagocytophila and Borrelia burgdorferi in Ixodes persulcatus ticks from northern China, *Am J Trop Med Hyg* 2003;68(5):547-50.

Christova, I, et al. High prevalence of granulocytic Ehrlichiae ad borrelia burgdorferi sensu lato in Ixodes ricinus ticks from Bulgaria, *J Clin Microbol* 2001;39(11):4172-4.

Derdakova, M, et al. Molecular evidence for Anaplasma phagocytophilum and Borrelia burgdorferi sensu lato in Ixodes ricinus ticks from eastern Slovakia, *Ann Agric Environ Med* 2003;10(2):269-71.

Hildebrandt, A. et al. Prevalence of four species of borrelia burgdorferi sensu lato and coinfection with Anaplasma phagocytophila in Ixodes ricinus ticks in central Germany, *Eur J Clin Microbiol Infect Dis* 2003;22(6):364-7.

Holden, K. et al. Detection of Borrelia burgdorferi, Ehrlichia chaffeensis, and Anaplasma phagocytophilum in ticks (Acari: Ixodidae) from a coastal region of California, *J Med Entomol* 2003;40(4):534-9.

Nochimson, Geofrey. Tick-Borne Diseases, Ehrlichiosis. Emedicine. www.emedicine.com. Accessed 2/1/2005.

Par, J and Rikihis, Y. L-arginine-dependent killing of intracellular Ehrlichia risticii by macrophages treated with gamma interferon, *Infect Immun* 1992;60(9);no page numbers avail.

Santino, I. et al. Multicentric study of seroprevalance of Borrelia burgdorferi and Anaplasma phagocytophila in high-risk groups in regions of central and southern Italy, *Int J Immunopathol Pharmacol* 2004;17(2):219-23.

Thomas, V, et al. Coinfection with Borreila burgdorferi and the agent of human granulocytic ehrlichiosis alters murine immune responses, pathogen burden, and severity of Lyme arthritis, *Infect Immun* 2001;69(5):3359-71.

Williams, J.C. and Kakoma, I., editors. *Ehrlichiosis*, Dordrect, The Netherlands:Kluwer Academic Publishers, 1990.

Zeidner, N.S. et al. Coinfection with Borrelia burgdorferi and the agent of human granulocytic ehrlichiosis suppresses IL-2 and IFN gamma production and promotes an IL-4 response in C3H/HeJ mice, *Parasite Immunol* 2000;22(11):581-8.

———. Transmission of the agent of human granulocytic ehrlichiosis by Ixodes spinipalpis ticks: evidence of an enzootic cycle of dual infection with Borrelia burgdorferi in Northern Colorado, *J Infect Dis* 2000;182(2):616-9.

HERBAL, GENERAL:

American Pharmaceutical Association. *The National Formulary*, Fourth Edition, Philadelphia, PA:Lippincott, 1916, Third Revision (1924).

Bensky, Dan and Gamble, Andrew. *Chinese Herbal Medicine Materia Medica*, Revised Edition, Seattle, Washington:Eastland Press, 1993.

Blumenthal, Mark, et al. *The Complete German Commission E Monographs*, Austin, TX: American Botanical Council, 1998.

Brown, O. Phelps. *The Complete Herbalist*, Jersey City, NJ: By the author, 1872.

Buhner, Stephen Harrod. *Herbal Antibiotics:Natural Alternatives for Treating Drug-resistant Bacteria*, Pownal, VT:Storey Publishing, 1999.

———. *Vital Man*, NY:Avery, 2003.

Chang, Hson-Mou and But, Paul Pui-Hay (eds). *Pharmacology and Applications of Chinese Materia Medica*, London:World Scientific, 1986, 2 vols.

Farquharson, Robert. *Guide to Therapeutics and Materia Medica*, Philadelphia, PA:Lea Brothers, 1889.

Felter and Lloyd, *King's American Dispensatory*, Sandy, Oregon: Eclectic Medical Publications, 1983 (1898), 2 vols.

Foster, Steven. *101 Medicinal Herbs*, Loveland, CO:Interweave Press, 1998.

——— and Chongxi, Yue. *Herbal Emissaries*, Rochester, VT:Healing Arts Press, 1992.

——— and Duke, James. *Eastern/Central Medicinal Plants* (Peterson Field Guide), Boston, MA:Houghton Mifflin, 1990.

Gladstar, Rosemary and Hirsch, Pamela, editors. *Planting the Future*, Rochester, VT:healing Arts Press, 2000.

Harborne, Jeffery, et al. *Phytochemical Dictionary*, Second Edition, London:Taylor and Francis, 1999.

Kuts-Chereaux, A.W. *Naturae Medicina and Naturopathic Dispensatory*, Des Moines, IA:American Naturopathic Physicians and Surgeons Associations, 1953.

Nadkarni, K.M. *Indian Materia Medica*, Third edition, Bombay:Popular Prakashan, 1954, 2 vols.

Pizzorno, Joseph and Murray, Michael. *Textbook of Natural Medicine*, Second Edition, NY:Churchill Livingstone, 1999, 2 vols.

Song, S. et al. Inhibitory effect of procyanidin oligomer from elm cortex on the matrix metalloproteinases and proteases of perodontopathogens, *Journal of Periodontal Research* 2003;38(3):282. "The procyanidin oligomer exhibited potent inhibitory effects on the MMPs in GCF (Mainly MMP-8 and -9) the pro and active forms of MMP-2 and trypsin-like enzymes from Treponema denticola."

Wood, Matthew. *The Book of Herbal Wisdom*, Berkeley, CA:North Atlantic Books, 1997.

Zhang, Y. et al. Fractionation and chemical properties of immuno-modulating polysaccharides from roots of Dipsacus asperoides, *Planta Med* 1997;63(5):393-9.

ANDROGRAPHIS:

Anonymous. Andrographis for the common cold. www.botanical pathways.com/issue10/Andro.html. Accessed 5/29/2004.

———. Andrographis paniculata: In-Depth review. http://altcancer.silvermedicine.org/an dcan.htm. Accessed 5/22/2004.

———. Paracelsian announces preliminary results of safety study show AndroVir(TM) will tolerated with decreases in HIV viral load and rapid increases in CD4 positive cells, PRnewswire, Thursday December 12, 1996. www.aegis.com/news/pr/1996. Accessed 11/23/2004.

Amaryan, G. et al. double-blind, placebo-controlled, randomized, pilot clinical trial of ImmunoGuard—a standardized fixed combination of Andrographis paniculata Nees, with Eleherococcus senticosus Maxim, Schizandra chinensis Bail. and Glycyrrhiza glabra L. extracts in patients with Familial Mediterranean Fever, *Phytomedicine* 2003;10(4): 271-85.

Balu, S. and Alagesaboothi, C. Anti-inflammatory activities of some species of Andrographis, *Ancient Science of Life* 1993;13:180-4.

Barilla, Jean. *Andrographis paniculata*, New Canaan, CT:Keats, 1999.

Batkuu, J. et al. Suppression of NO production in activated macrophages in vitro and ex vivo by neoandrographolide isolated from Andrographis paniculata, *Biol Pharm Bull* 2002;25(9):1169-74.

Calabrese, C. et al. A phase I trial of andrographolide in HIV positive patients and normal volunteers, *Phytother Res* 2000;14(5):333-8.

Chaturvedi, G. et al. Clinical studies on Kalmegh (Andrographis paniculata) in infective hepatitis, *Ancient Sci Life* 1983;2:208.

Chauhan, C. et al. effect of a herbal hepatoprotective product on drug metabolism in patients of cirrhosis and hepatic enzyme function in experimental liver damage, *Ind J Pharmacol* 1992;24:107-10.

Deng, W. Pharmacological studies on 13 kinds of injections from Andrographis paniculata: antipyretic, anti-inflammatory effects and toxicity, *Chung Yao Tung Pao* 1985;10:38-42.

Duke, James. Chemicals and Their Biological Activities in Andrographis paniculata (BURM, f.) NEES (Acanthaceae). www.ars-grin.gov/cgi-bin/duke. Accessed 11/24/2004.

Dutta, A. and Sukul N. Filariasis properties of a wild herb, Andrographis paniculata, *J Helminthol* 1982;56:81-84.

Gabrielian, E. et al A double-blind, placebo-controlled study of Andrographis paniculata fixed combination Kan Jang in the treatment of acute upper respiratory tract infections including sinusitis, *Phytomedicine* 2002;9(7):589-97.

Gupta, S. et al. Antisecretory (anti-diarrheal) activity of Indian medicinal plants against E. coli induced secretion in rabbit and guinea pig ileal loop models, *Int J Pharmacognosy* 1993;31:198-204.

Hancke, J. et al. A double-blind study with a new monodrug Kan Jang:decrease of symptoms and improvements in the recovery from common colds, *Phytotherapy Res* 1995;(no journal number available):559-62.

Huo, T. and Jinzhi, T. Study on antiplatelet aggregation effect of Andrographis paniculata, *Chinese Journal of Integrated Traditional and Western Medicine* 1989;9:540-2.

Koul, I. and Kapil, A. Effect of diterpenes from Andrographis paniculata on antioxidant defense system and lipid peroxidation, *Indian Journal of Pharmacology* 1994;26(4):296-300.

Madav, S. et al. Analgesic, antipyretic, and antiulcerogenic effects of andrographolide, *Indian Journal of Pharmaceutical Sciences* 1995;57(3):121-5.

Madhav, S. et al. Antiallergenic activity of andrographolide, *Indian Journal of Pharmaceutical Sciences* 1998;60(3):176-8.

Melchior, J. et al. Double-blind, placebo-controlled pilot and phase III study of activity of standardized Andrographis paniculata herba Nees extract fixed combination (Kan Jang) in the treatment of uncomplicated upper-respiratory tract infection, *Phytomedicine* 2000;7(5):341-50.

Misra, P. Antimalarial activity of Andrographis paniculata (Kalmegh) against Plasmodium NK65 in Mastomys natalensis, *Int J Pharmacol* 1992;30:263-74.

Nanduri, S. et al. Anticancer compounds: processes for their preparation and pharmaceutical compositions containing them, *United States Patents* 6,410,590 and 6,486,196 and 6,576,662, June 25, 2002, November 26, 2002, and June 10, 2003.

Panossian, A. et al. Effect of andrographolide and Kan Jan—fixed combination of extract SHA-10 and extract SHE-3—on proliferation of human lymphocytes, production of cytokines and immune activation markers in the whole blood cells culture, *Phytomedicine* 2002;9(7): 598-605.

Peng, G. et al. Modulation of lianbizi injection (andrographolide) on some immune functions, *Zhongguo Zhong Yao Za Zhi* 2002;27(2):147-50.

Raj, R. Screening of indigenous plants for anthelmintic actions against Ascaris lumbricoids: Part II, *Ind J Physiol Pharmacol* 1975;19:no page numbers available.

Rajagopal, S. et al. Andrographolide, a potential cancer therapeutic agent isolated from Andrographis paniculata, *J Exp Ther Oncol* 2003;3(3):147-58.

Rao, T. et al. Observations on the reduction of sotha in cases of slipada (filariasis) with Nityanandaras and Bhunumba vati- a pilot study, *J Ayur Siddha* 1985;6(1,3,4):59-77.

Shahid, A. Anti-inflammatory activity of Andrographis paniculata Nees (Chirayata), *Hamdard Medicus* 1987;30:63-9.

Shakhova, E. et al. Effectiveness of using the drug Kan-Yang in children with acute respiratory viral infection (clinico-functional data), *Vestn Ororinolaringol* 2003;3:48-50.

Sinja, J. et al. Targeting of liposomal andrographolide to L. donovani-infected macrophages in vivo, *Drug Deliv* 2000;7(4):209-13.

Siti, M. et al. The screening of extracts from Goniothalamus scortechinii, Aralidum pinnatifidum and Andrographis paniculata for anti-malarial activity using the lactate dehydrogenase assay, *J Ethnopharmacol* 2002;82(2):239-42.

Srivastava, V. and Tandon, J. Immunostimulant agents from Andrographis paniculata, *J Nat Products* 1993;56:995-9.

Tajuddin, S. and Tariq, M. Anti-inflammatory activity of Andrographis paniculata Nees (Chirayata), *Nagarjun* 1983;27:13-14.

Wang, T. et al. Andrographolide reduces inflammation-mediated dopaminergic neurodegeneration in mesencephalic neuron-glial cultures by inhibiting microglial activation, *J Pharmacol Exp Ther* 2004;308(3):975-83.

Wen-fei, C. et al. Anti-inflammatory effect of andographolide [sic]: suppression of C5a-induced chemotactic migration and evaluating the role of different intracellular signal pathways, *12th International Conference on Oriental Medicine* 2003;0-35.

Zhang, C. and Tan, B. Hypotensive activity of aqueous extract of Andrographis paniculata in rats, *Clin Exp Pharmacol Physiol* 1997;23:675-8.

———. Mechanics of cardiovascular activity of Andrographis paniculata in the anesthetized rat, *J Ethnopharmacol* 1997;56:97-101.

Zhao, H. and Fang, W. Combined Chinese and western medicine— antithrombotic effects of Andrographis paniculata Nees in preventing myocardial infarction, *Chinese Medical Journal* 1991;104:770-5.

Zhi-ling, G. et al. Effect of Andrographis paniculata extract on intracellular electrolytes in cardiac ischemia reperfusion, *Chinese J Pathophysiology* 1992;10:591-4.

Zhong, H. et al. Investigation of M, N, and T antigenic components in Chinese medicinal herbs, *Kexne Tongbao* 1982:27:112-5.

ARTEMISIA:

Allen, P. et al. Effects of components of Artemisia annua on coccidia infections in chickens, *Poult Sci* 1997;76(8):1156-63.

Chen, H. et al. Inhibitory effects of artesunate on angiogenesis and on expressions of vascular endothelial growth factor and VEGF receptor KDR/flk-1, *Pharmacology* 2004;71(1): 1-9.

Dharmananda, Subhuti. Qing-hao and the artemisias used in Chinese medicine. www.canmedbotanics.nl/art.htm. Accessed 12/12/2004.

Duke, James. Chemicals and their biological effects in Artemisia annua L. (Asteraceae). www.ars-grin.gov. Accessed 12/12/2004.

Eckstein-Ludwig, U. et al. Artemisinins target the SERCA of Plasmodium falciparum, *Nature* 2003;424(6951): 957-61.

Ferreira, J. and Janick, J. Distribution of artemisinin in Artemisia annua, in Janick, editor, *Progress in New Crops*, Arlington, VA:ASHS Press, 1996, ppg 579-84.

Gordi, T. Clinical Pharmacokinetics of the Antimalarial Artemisinin Based on Saliva Sampling, Doctoral Thesis, 2001.

——— et al. Artemisinin pharmacokinetics and efficacy in uncomplicated malaria patients treated with two different dosage regimens, *Antimicrob Agents Chemother* 2002;46(4):1026-31.

Hatimi, S. et al. In vitro evaluation of antileishmania activity of Artemisia herba alba Asso, *Bull Soc Pathol Exot* 2001;94(1):29-31.

Huan-huan, C. et al. Artesunate reduces chicken chorioallantoic membrane neovascularization and exhibits antiangiogenic and apoptotic activity on human microvascular dermal endothelial cell, *Cancer Lett* 2004;211(2):163-73.

Huang, L. et al. Antipyretic and anti-inflammatory effects of Artemisia annua L., *Zhongguo Zhong Yao Za Zhi* 1993;18(1):44-8, 63-4.

Jung, M. et al. Recent advances in artemisinin and its derivatives as antimalarial and antitumor agents, *Curr Med Chem* 2004;11(10):1265-84.

Kim, J. et al. In vitro antiprotozoal effects of artemisinin on Neospora caninum, *Vet Parasitol* 202;103(1-2): 53-63.

Mueller, M. et al. Randomized controlled trial of a traditional preparation of Artemisia annua L. (annual wormwood) in the treatment of malaria, *Trans R Soc Med Hyg* 2004;98(5):318-21.

Puotinen, C. Artemisinin, Malaria, and Cancer, NEHA Journal, Winter 2003, no page numbers available.

Rath, K. et al. Pharmakokinetic study of artemisinin after oral intake of a traditional preparation of Artemisia annua L. (annual wormwood), *Am J Trop Med hyg* 2004;70(2):128-32.

Shuhua, X. et al. Preventive effect of artemether in experimental animals infected with Schistosoma mansoni, *Parasitol Int* 2000;49(1):19-24.

Singh, N. and Lai, H. Artemisinin induces apoptosis in human cancer cells, *Anticancer Res* 2004;24(4): 2277-80.

Stermitz, F. et al. Two flavonols from Artemisia annua which potentiate the activity of berberine and norfloxacin against a resistant strain of Staphylococcus aureus, *Planta Med* 2002;68(12):1140-1.

Tan, Y. et al. Experimental study on antiendotoxin effect of extracts from Artemisia annua L., *Zhongguo Zhong Yao Za Zhi* 1999;24(3):166-71.

Tawfik, A. et al. Effects of artemisinin, dihydroartemisinin and artemether on immune responses of normal mice, *Int J Immunopharmacol* 1990;12(4):385-9.

Townsend Letter. Artemisinin: Malaria to Cancer Treatment. www.townsendletter.com/Dec2002/ artemisinin1202.htm. Accessed 12/12/2004.

Wang, Q. et al. Experimental studies of antitumor effect of artesunate on liver cancer, *Zhongguo Zhong Yao Za Zhi* 2001;26(10):707-8, 720.

Wong, J. et al. Therapeutic equivalence of a low dose artemisinin formulation in falciparum malaria patients, *Journal of Pharmacy and Pharmacology* 2003;55(2):193.

ASTRAGALUS:

Anonymous. Astragalus membranaceus (Fisch.). www.herbmed.org. Accessed 12/25/2004.

Chen, K. et al. Reducing fatigue of athletes following oral administration of huangqi jianzhong tang, *Acta Pharmacol Sin* 2002;23(8):757-61.

Chen, L. et al. Effects of Astragalus membranaceus on left ventricular function and oxygen free radical in acute myocardial infarction patients and mechanism of its cardiotonic action, *Zhongguo Zhong Xi Jie He Za Zhi* 1995;15(3):141-3.

Duan, P. and Wang, Z. Clinical study on effect of Astragalus in efficacy enhancing and toxicity reducing of chemotherapy in patients of malignant tumor, *Zhongguo Zhong Xi Jie He Za Zhi* 2002;22(7):515-7.

Duke, James. Chemicals in Astragalus membranaceus (Fisch.Ex Link) Bunge (Fabaceae). www.ars-grin.gov. Accessed 12/31/2004.

Li, S. et al. Clinical observation on the treatment of ischemic heart disease with Astragalus membranaceus, *Zhongguo Zhong Xi Jie He Za Zhi* 1995;15(2):77.

Li, Z. et al. Effect of astragalus injection on immune function in patients with congestive heart failure, *Zhongguo Zhong Xi Jie He Za Zhi* 2003;23(5):351-3.

———. Effect of milkvetch injection on immune function of children with tetralogy of Fallot after radical operation, *Zhongguo Zhong Xi Jie He Za Zhi* 2004;24(7):596-600.

Luo, H. et al. Nuclear cardiology study on effective ingredients of Astragalus membranaceus in treating heart failure, *Zhongguo Zhong Xi Jie He Za Zhi* 1995;15(12):707-9.

Mao, S. et al. Modulatory effect of Astragalus membranaceus on Th1/Th2 cytokine in patients with herpes simplex keratitis, *Zhongguo Zhong Xi Jie He Za Zhi* 2004;24(2):121-3.

Shi, H. et al. Primary research on the clinical significance of ventricular late potentials (VLPs), and the impact of mexiletine, lidocaine and Astragalus membranaceus on VLPs, *Zhongguo Zhong Xi Jie He Za Zhi* 1991;11(5):265-7, 259.

Wei, H. Traditional Chinese medicine Astragalus reverses predominance of Th2 cytokines and their up-stream transcript factors in lung cancer patients, *Oncol Rep* 2003;10(5): 1507-12.

COLCHICUM:

Adhami, J. and Basho, J. Treatment with colchicine and survival of patients with ascitic cirrhoses: a double-blind randomized trial, *Panminerba Med* 1998;40(1):75-9.

Anonymous. Colchicine Drug Information. 26 pages. www.drugs.com. Accessed 10/31/2004.

Akar, A. et al. Efficacy and safety assessment of .05% and 1% colchicine cream in the treatment of actinic keratoses, *J Dermatolog Treat* 2001;12(4):199-203.

Banodkar, D. and al-Suwaid, A. Colchicine as a novel therapeutic agent in chronic bulbous dermatosis of childhood, *Int J Dermatol* 1997;36(3):213-6.

Bemer, V. et al. Colchicum autumnale agglutin activates all murine T-lymphocytes but does not induce the proliferation of all activated cells, *Cell Immunol* 1996;172(1):60-9.

Cacoub, P. et al. Efficacy of colchicine in recurrent acute idiopathic pericarditis, *Arch Mal Coeur Vaiss* 2000;93(12):1511-4.

Das, S. et al. A randomized controlled trial to evaluate the slow-acting symptom-modifying effects of colchicine in osteoarthritis of the knee: a preliminary report, *Arthritis Rheum* 2002; 47(3): 280-4.

Dubois, R. et al. Regulation of gelatinase B (MMP-9) in leukocytes by plant lectins, *FEBS Lett* 1998;427(2):275-8.

Duke, James. Activities of Colchicine, *Phytochemical and Ethnobotanical Database.* www.ars-grin.gov. Accessed 10/31/2004.

————. Chemicals in Colchicum autumnale, *Phytochemical and Ethnobotanical Database.* www.ars-grin.gov. Accessed 10/31/2004.

Finkelstein, Y. et al. Colchicine for the prevention of postpericardiotomy syndrome, *Herz* 2002;27(8):791-4.

Fontes, V. et al. Recurrent aphthous stomatitis: treatment with colchicine. An open trial of 54 cases, *Ann Dermatol Venererol* 2002;129(12):1365-9.

Frame, P. et al. Use of colchicine to treat severe constipation in developmentally disabled patients, *J Am Board Fam Pract* 1998; 11(5):341-6.

Go, R. et al. Human cyclic thrombocytopenia and Anaplasma spp infection, *Eur J Haemotology* 2005;74)2):182-3.

Kaplan, M. et al. A randomized controlled trial of colchicine plus ursodiol versus methotrexate plus ursodiol in primary biliary cirrhosis: ten year results, *Hepatology* 2004;39(4):915-23.

Kelly, S. et al. Effects of colchicine on IgE-mediated early and late airway reactions, *Chest* 1995;107(4):985-91.

Kiraz, S. et al. Effects of colchicine on inflammatory cytokines and selectins in familial Mediterranean fever, *Clin Exp Rheumatol* 1998;16(6):721-4.

Lascaratos, J. "Arthritis" in Byzantium (AD 324-1453)" unknown information from non-medical literary sources, *Ann Rheum Dis* 1995; 54(12):951-7.

Li, W. et al. Effects of da ding feng zhu decoction in 30 cases of liver fibrosis, *J Trad Chin Med* 2003;23(4):251-4.

McColm, A. et al. Inhibition of malaria parasite invasion into erythrocytes pretreated with membrane-active drugs, *Mol Biochem Parasitol* 1980;1(2):119-27.

Monti, G. et al. Colchicine in the treatment of mixed cryoglobulinemia, *Clin Exp Rheumatol* 1995;13(Supp 13):S197-9.

Myrhed, M. Uric acid and arthritis in Australia. Purified plant extract from meadow saffron is a good preparation against acute gout attacks, *Lakartidningen* 1982;79(19):1893-4.

Prieto, R. et al. Combined treatment with vitamin E and colchicine in the early stages of Peyronie's disease, *BJU Int* 2003;91(6):522-4.

Rikihisa, Y. et al. Inhibition of infection of macrophages with Ehrlichia risticii by cytochalasins, monodany-sylcadaverine, and taxol, *Infect Immun* 1994;62(11):5126-32.

Sais, G. et al. Colchicine in the treatment of cutaneous leukocytoclastic vasculitis. Results of a prospective, randomized controlled trial. *Arch Dermatol* 1995;13(12):1399-402.

Tuzun, F. et al. Multicenter, randomized, double-blinded, placebo-controlled trial of thiocolchicoside in acute low back pain, *Joint Bone Spine* 2003;70(5):356-61.

Verne, G. et al. Colchicine is an effective treatment for patients with chronic constipation: an open-label trial, *Dig Dis Sci* 1997; 42(9):1959-63.

————— et al. Treatment of chronic constipation with colchicine: randomized, double-blind, placebo-controlled, crossover trial, *Am J Gastroenterol* 2003;98(5):1112-6.

Yurdakul, S. et al. A double-blind trial of colchicine in Behcet's syndrome, *Arthritis Rheum* 2001;44(11):2686-92.

POLYGONUM CUSPIDATUM:

Anonymous. Several Chinese medicinal herbal extracts are strong angiogenesis modulators, May 6, 2004. www.merckmedicus.com (NewsRx.com). Accessed 5/30/2004.

Cavazza, Claudio. Combination of carnitines and resveratrol for prevention or treatment of cerebral and aging disorders, *United States Patent* 6,515,020, February 4, 2003.

Ching-jer, C. et al. Oncogene signal transduction inhibitors from Chinese medicinal plants, *Pure Appl Chem* 1999;71(6):1101-4.

Docherty, J. Method of inhibiting formation of infectious microorganisms, *United States Patent*, 6,355,692, March 12, 2002.

Docherty, J. et al. Resveratrol selectively inhibits Neisseria gonorhoeae and Neisseria meningitidis, *Journal of Antimicrobial Chemotherapy* 2001;47:243-44.

Egemen, S. et al. Red wine ingredient resveratrol protects from B-amyloid neurotoxicity, *Gerontology* 2003;49: 380-3.

English, J. Resveratrol mimics caloric restriction to turn on "longevity genes." *VRP Newsletter*, October 2003, no page numbers.

Feng, Y. et al. Low dose resveratrol enhanced immune response of mice, *Acta Pharmacol Sin* 2002;23(10): 893-7.

Gupta, Y. et al. Effect of trans resveratrol on ischemia reperfusion induced by middle cerebral artery occlusion in rats, *Life Sci* 2002;71(21):2489-98.

Hao, H. and He, L. New progression in the study of protective properties of resveratrol in cardiovascular disease, *Bratisl Lek Listy* 2004;105(5-6):225-9.

Hegde, V. et al. Two new bacterial DNA primase inhibitors from the plant Polygonum cuspidatum, *Bioorg Med Chem Lett* 2004;14(9):2275-7.

Hensley, Kenneth, et al. Method for using tethered bis(polyhydroxy-phenyls) and O-alkyl derivatives thereof in treating inflammatory conditions of the central nervous system, *United States Patent* 20040014721, January 22, 2004.

Howitz, K. et al. Small molecule activators of sirtuins extend saccharomyces cerevisiae lifespan, *Nature* 2003;425(6954):191-6.

Ignatowicz, E. and Baer-Dubowska, W. Resveratrol, a natural chemopreventative agent against degenerative diseases, *Polish Journal of Pharmacology* 2001;53:557-69.

Karlsson, J. et al. Trans-resveratrol protects embryonic mesencephalic cells from tert-butyl hydroperoxide: electron paramagnetic resonance spin trapping evidence for a radical scavenging mechanism, *Journal of Neurochemistry* 2000;75:141-50.

Kimura, Y. and Okuda, H. resveratrol isolated rom Polygonum cuspidatum root prevents tumor growth and metastasis to lung and tumor-induced neovascularization in Lewis lung carcinoma-bearing mice, *J Nutr* 2001;131(6):1844-9.

Leiro, J. et al. Resveratrol modulates rat macrophage functions, *Int Immunopharmacol* 2002;2(6):767-74.

Li, Y. et al. Inhibition of dexamethasone, indomethacinand resveratrol on matrix metalloproteinase-9 and the mechanism of inhibition, *Yao Xue Xue Bao* 2003;38(7):501-4.

———— et al. Resveratrol inhibits matrix metalloproteinase-9 transcription in U937 cells, *Acta Pharmacol Sin* 2003;24(11):1167-71.

Lin, S. Rein inhibits TPA-induced activator protein-1 activation and cell transformation by blocking the JNK-dependent pathway, *Int J Oncol* 2003;22(4):829-33.

Meishiang, J. and Pezzuto, J. Resveratrol blocks eicosanoid production and chemically-induced cellular transformation: implications for cancer chemoprevention, *Pharmaceutical Biology* 1998;36:28-34.

Ming-Tsan, L. et al. Inhibition of vascular endothelial growth factor-induced angiogenesis by resveratrol through interruption of src-dependent vascular endothelial cadherin tyrosine phosphorylation, *Mol Pharmacol* 2003;64:1029-36.

Nicolini, G. et al. Anti-apoptotic effect of trans-resveratrol on paclitaxel-induced apoptosis in the human neuroblastoma SH-SY5Y cell line, *Neurosci Lett* 2001;302(1):41-4.

Park, C. et al. Inhibitory effects of Polygonum cuspidatum water extract (PCWE) and its component resveratrol on acyl-coenzyme A-cholesterol acyltransferase activity for cholesteryl ester synthesis in HepG2 cells, *Vascul Pharmacol* 2004; 49(6): 279-84.

Pervaiz, S. Resveratrol: from grapevines to mammalian biology, *The FASEB Journal* 2003;17:1975-85.

Pinto, M. et al. Resveratrol is a potent inhibitor of the dioxygenase activity of lipoxygenase, *J Agric Food Chem* 1999;47(12):4842-6.

Rotondo, S. et al. Effect of trans-resveratrol, a natural polyphenolic compound, in human polymorpho-nuclear leukocyte function, *Br J Pharmacol* 1998;123(8):1691-9.

Roug, Y. et al. Resveratrol inhibits phorbol ester and UV-induced activator protein 1 activation by interfering with mitogen-activated protein kinase pathways, *Molecular Pharmacology* 2001;60(1): 217-24.

Schroecksnadel, K. et al. Resveratrol modulates interferon-y-induced neopterin production and tryptophan degradation in human PBMC, *ICI/Focis 2004 Abstracts*. www.immuno2004.org/ onlineabstracts/bycategory/37.html. Accessed 2/05/05.

Sharma, M. and Gupta, Y. Chronic treatment with trans resveratrol prevents intracerebroventricular streptozotocin induced cognitive impairment and oxidative stress in rats, *Life Sci* 2002;71(21):2489-98.

Shuang-Cheng, M. et al. Antiviral Chinese medicinal herbs against respiratory syncytial virus, *Journal of Ethnopharmacology* 2002; 79:205-11.

Smolarz, H. et al. Influence of ethyl acetate extract and quercetin-3-methyl ether from Polygonum amphibium on activation lymphocytes from peripheral blood of healthy donor in vitro, *Phytother Res* 2003;17(7):744-7.

Spainhour, J. Medical Attributes of *Polygonum cuspidatum*—Japanese Knotweed, July 1997. http://wilkes1. wilkes.edu/~kklemow/Polygonum. html. Accessed 5/30/2004.

Tegos, G. et al. Multidrug pump inhibitors uncover remarkable activity of plant antimicrobials, *Antimicrobial Agents and Chemotherapy* 2002;46(10):3133-41.

Tong, W. et al. The mechanisms of lipoxygenase inhibitor-induced apoptosis in human breast cancer cells, *Biochem Biophys res Commun* 2002;296(4):942-8.

Usha, R. et al. Resveratrol, a polyphenolic compound found in wine, inhibits tissue factor expression in vascular cells, *Arteriosclerosis, Thrombosis, and Vascular Biology* 1999;19:419-26.

Williams, R. et al. Polyphenolic phytoestrogenic agents: their biological activity in human cancer cell studies, *2nd International Electronic Conference on Synthetic Organic Chemistry* September 1-30, 1998. www.mdpi.org/ecsos/. Accessed 2/05/05.

Woo, J. et al. Resveratrol inhibits phorbol myristate acetate-induced matrix metalloproteinase-9 expression by inhibiting JNK and PKC delta signal transduction, *Oncogene* 2004;23(10): 1845-53.

Yang, Y. and Piao, Y. Effects of resveratrol on secondary damages after acute spinal cord injury in rats, *Acta Pharmacol Sin* 2003;24(7):703-10.

Zhao, K. et al. The mechanism of Polydatin in shock treatment, *Clin Hemorheol Microcirc* 2003;29(3-4): 211-7.

SMILAX:

Chen, T. et al. A new flavone isolated from rhizoma Smilacis glabrae and the structure requirements of its derivatives for preventing immunological hepatocyte damage, *Planta Med* 1999;65(1):56-9.

Diaz, L. et al. Comparative study between "First Call," a complex of flavinoids and polyphenols created from extracts of artichoke and sarsaparilla, and placebo in alcohol related liver disease, 2003. www.naturalbridges.ws/full_study. html. Accessed 2/6/2005.

Duke, James. Chemicals and their Biological Activities in Smilax spp (Smilacaceae)—Sarsaparilla. www.ars-grin.gov. Accessed 11/30/2004.

Fitzpatrick, F. Plant substances active against mycobacterium tuberculosis, *Antibiotics and Chemotherapy* 1954;4(5):528-36.

Jiang, J. and Xu, Q. Immunomodulatory activity of the aqueous extract rom rhizome of Smilax glabra in the later phase of adjuvant-induced arthritis in rats, *J Ethnopharmacol* 2003;85(1): 53-9.

Lee, S. et al. Free radical scavenging and antioxidant enzyme fortifying activities of extracts from Smilax china root, *Exp Mol Med* 2001;33(4):263-8.

Lu, Y. et al. Effect of Smilax china on adjunctive arthritis mouse, *Zhong Yao Cai* 2003;26(5):344-6.

Navarro, M. et al. Antibacterial, antiprotozoal, and antioxidant activity of five plants used in Izabal for infectious diseases, *Phytother Res* 2003;17(4):325-9.

Panda, H. *Handbook on Herbal Drugs and Its Plant Sources,* Delhi:INdia:National Institute of Industrial Research, 2004.

Rafatullah, S. et al. Hepatoprotective and safety evaluation studies on sarsaparilla, *Int J Pharmacognosy* 1991;29:296-301.

Rhee, J. et al. Screening of the wormicidal Chinese raw drugs on Clonorchis sinensis, *Am J Chin Med* 1981;9(4):277-84.

Roller, R. et al. An extract of Smilax ornata corresponding to 15g of root given twice a day for several months gave better results in lepers than did sulfones, *Maroc Med* 1951;30:776-80.

Stout, Timothy. Speculation Concerning Lyme Disease, MS, and Sarsaparilla. www.el-dorado.ca.us/~tstout/articles. Accessed 5/8/2004.

Tanaka, M. et al. Therapeutic agents for respiratory diseases, *United States Patent* 6,309, 674, October 30, 2001.

Taylor, Leslie. *Technical Data Report for Sarsaparilla; Smilax officinalis*, Austin, TX:Sage Press, 2003.

Xia, et al. Smilagenin and its use, *United States Patent* 6,258,386, July 10, 2001.

———. Steroidal sapogenins and their derivatives for treating Alzheimer's disease, *United States Patent* 6,812, 213, November 2, 2004.

Xu, et al. Immunosuppressive agents, *United States Patent* 6,531,505, March 11, 2003.

Yi, Y. et al. Studies on the chemical constituents of Smilax glabra, *Yao Xue Xue Bao* 1998;33(11):873-5.

Zhamg, et al. Smilax, diabetes, and urinary tract infections, *Zhong Yi Za Zhi* 2001;12:713.

STEPHANIA:

Anonymous. Stephania Root. www.holistic-online.com. Accessed 12/31/04.

Chang, M. et al. The influence of Chinese traditional medicine on the production and activity of interleukin I (IL-I), *Zhonghua Min Guo Wei Shend Wu Ji Mian Yi Xue Za Zhi* 1993;26(1):15-24.

CHoi, H. et al. Anti-inflammatory effects of fangchinoline and tetrandrine, *J Ethnopharmacol* 2000;69(2):173-9.

Cunningham, Dean. Quenching the flames of inflammation, *Life Extension Magazine*, July 2004, no page numbers available.

Derrida, Michael. Tetrandrine. www.newigwam.com. Accessed 1/2/05.

Ding-Guo, L. et al. Pharmacology of tetrandrine and its therapeutic use in digestive diseases, *World J Gastronenterol* 2001;7(5):627-9.

Duke, James. Chemicals and their Biological Activities in Stephania tetrandra. www.ars-grin.gov. Accessed 12/19/04.

Ferrante, A. et al. Tetrandrine, a plant alkaloid, inhibits the production of tumor necrosis factor-alpha (cachectin) by human monocytes, *Clin Exp Immunol* 1990;80(2):232-5.

Fu L. et al. Characterization of tetrandrine, a potent inhibitor of P-glycoprotein-mediated multidrug resistance, *Cancer Chemother Pharmacol* 2004;53(4):349-56.

Ho, L and Lai J. Chinese herba as immunomodulators and potential disease-modifying antirheumatic drugs in autoimmune disorders, *Curr Drug Metab* 2004;5(2):181-92.

Hu, S. et al. Comparative effectiveness and molecular pharmacological mechanisms of antiallergic agents on experimental conjunctivitis in mice, *J Ocul Pharmacol Ther* 1998;14(1):67-74.

Kobayashi, S. et al. Inhibitory effects of tetrandrine and related synthetic compounds on angiogenesis in streptozocin-diabetic rodents, *Biol Pharm Bull* 1999;22(4):360-5.

Koh, S. et al. Protective effects of fangchinoline and tetrandrine on hydrogen peroxide-induced oxidative neuronal cell damage in cultured rat cerebellar granule cells, *Planta Med* 2003;69(6):506-12.

Kosuke, J. et al. Potent enhancement of the sensitivity of Plasmodium falciparum to chloroquine by the bisbenzylisoquinoline alkaloid cepharanthin, *Antimicrobial Agents and Chemotherapy* 2000;44(10):2706-8.

Lai, J. Immunomodulatory effects and mechanisms of plant alkaloid tetrandrine in autoimmune diseases, *Acta Pharmacol Sin* 2002;23(12):1093-101.

Li, S. et al. Anti-inflammatory and immunosuppressive properties of bis-benzulisoquinolines: in vitro comparisons of tetrandrine and berbamine, *Int J Immunopharmacol* 1989;11(4):395-401.

Liang, X. et al. Therapeutic efficacy of Stephania tetrandra S. Moore for treatment of neovascularization of retinal capillary (retinopathy) in diabetes—in vitro study, *Phytomedicine* 1002;9(5):377-84.

Liu, D. et al. Effects of tetrandrine on the synthesis of collagen and scar-derived fibroblast DNA, *Zhonghua Shao Shang Za Zhi* 2001; 17(4):222-4.

Liu, S. et al. Effects of Chinese herbal products on mammalian retinal functions, *J Ocul Pharmacol Ther* 1996;12(3):377-86.

Lu, Y. Clinical observation on the termination of paroxysmal supraventricular tachycardia by tetrandrine, *Zhongua Xin Xue Guan Za Zhi* 1990;18(3):164-5.

Niizawa, A. et al. Clinical and immunomodulatory effects of funboi, an herbal medicine, on collagen-induced arthritis in vivo, *Clin Exp Rheumatol* 2003;21(1):57-62.

Okamoto, M. et al. Suppression of cytokine production and neural cell death by the anti-inflammatory alkaloid cepharanthine: a potential agent against HIV-1 encephalopathy, *Biochem Pharmacol* 2001;62(6):747-53.

Rao, M. Effects of tetrandrine on cardiac and vascular remodeling, *Acta Pharmacol Sin* 2002;23(12):1075-85.

Seow, W. et al. Antiphagocytic and antioxidant properties of plant alkaloid tetrandrine, *Int Arch Allergy Appl Immunol* 1988;85(4):404-9.

———. In vitro immunosuppressive properties of the plant alkaloid tetrandrine, *Int Arch Allergy Appl Immunol* 1988;85(4):410-5.

———. Inhibitory effects of tetrandrine on human neutrophil and monocyte adherence, *Immunol Lett* 1986;13(1-2):83-8.

Shen, E. et al. Anti-inflammatory effects of the partially purified extract of radix Stephaniae tetrandrae: comparative studies of its active principles tetrandrine and fangchinoline on human polymorphonuclear leukocyte functions, *Mol Pharmacol* 2001;60(5):1083-90.

The, B. et al. Inhibition of prostaglandin and leukotriene generation by the plant alkaloids tetrandrine and berbamine, *Int J Immunopharmacol* 1990;12(3):321-6.

Tsai, J. et al. The modulatory effect of tetrandrine on the CD23, CD25 and HLA-DR expression and cytokine production in different groups of asthmatic patients, *Int Arch Allergy Immunol* 1995;108(2):183-8.

Wiegand, H. et al. Inhibition by tetrandrine of calcium currents at mouse motor nerve endings, *Brain Res* 1990;524(1):112-8.

Wong, C. et al. Comparative immunopharmacology and toxicology of the bisbenzyliso-quinoline alkaloids tetrandrine and berbamine, *Int J Immunopharmacol* 1991;13(5):579-85.

Wong, T. et al. Cardiovascular actions of Radix Stephaniae Tetrandrae: a comparison with its main component, tetrandrine, *Acta Pharmacol Sin* 2000;21(12):1083-8.

Yao, W. and Jiang, M. Effects of tetrandrine on cardiovascular electrophysiologic properties, *Acta Pharmacol Sin* 2002;23(12):1069-74.

Xiao, J and Chiou, G. Tetrandrine inhibits breakdown of blood-aqueous barrier induced by endotoxin and interleukin-1 alpha in rats, *J Ocul Pharmacol Ther* 1996;12(3):323-9.

Xie, Q. et al. Pharmacological actions of tetrandrine in inflammatory pulmonary diseases, *Acta Pharmacol Sin* 2002;23(12)1107-13.

Zeng, B. and Dai, G. Effect of tetrandrine and verapamil on left ventricular diastolic and systolic function in essential hypertension, *Zhonghua Nei Ke Za Zhi* 1991;30(3):134-7,187.

UNCARIA:

Aguilar, J. et al. Anti-inflammatory activity of two different extracts of Uncaria tomentosa (Rubiaceae), *J Ethnopharmacol* 2002;81(2):271-6.

Akesson, C. et al. C-Med-100, a hot water extract of Uncaria tomentosa, prolongs lymphocyte survival in vivo, *Phytomedicine* 2003;10(1):23-33.

———. An extract of Uncaria tomentosa inhibiting cell division and NF-kappa B activity without inducing cell death, *Int Immunopharmacol* 2003;3(13-14):1889-1900.

Allergy Research Group, Prima Una de Gato, September 2003, product description sheet.

Bazyka, D. et al. Manaxx, lyphophilized extract of Uncaria tomentosa (Willd.), in clinical immunology after radiation exposure, Research Center of Radiation Medicine (Kiev, Ukraine). www.manaxx.com/estudios-e1.htm. Accessed 11/26/2004.

Bednarek, D. et al. Analysis of phenotype and functions of peripheral blood leukocytes in cellular immunity of calves treated with Uncaria tomentosa, *Bull Vet Inst Pulawy* 2004;48:289-296.

———. Modulating effects of Uncaria tomentosa in experimentally-induced local pneumonia in calves, *Bull Vet Inst Pulawy* 2002;46:65-77.

Castillo, G. and Snow, A. Methods for inhibiting and reducing amyloid fibril formation associated with Alzheimer's disease and other amyloidoses, *United States Patent* 6,607,758, August 19, 2003.

Cowden, W. et al. Pilot study of pentacyclic alkaloid-chemotype of Uncaria tomentosa for the treatment of Lyme disease, December 28-2002-March 22, 2003. Presented at the International Symposium for Natural Treatment of Intracellular Micro Organisms (March 29, 2003) Munich, Germany. also: Lyme disease: Nutraceutical breakthrough using TOA-free cat's claw (Prima una de gato): study shows pentacyclic alkaloid chemotype Uncaria tomentosa to be effective in treating Chronic Lyme disease (Lyme borreliosis). www.springboard4health.com. Accessed 1/5/2005)

Deharo, E. et al. In vitro immuno-modulatory activity of plants used by the Tacana ethnic group in Bolivia, *Phytomedicine* 2004;11(6):516-22.

Falkiewicz, B. and Lukasiak, J. Vilacora [Uncaria tomentosa (Willd.) DC. and Uncaria guianensis (Aublet0 Gmell.]—a review of published scientific literature, *Case Rep Clin Prac Rev* 2001;2(4):305-16.

Goto, H. et al. Effect of Uncariae ramulus et Uncus on endothelium in spontaneously hypertensive rats, *Am J Chin Med* 1999;27(3):339-45.

Harada, M et al. Ganglion blocking effect of indole alkaloids contained in Uncaria genus and Amsonia genus and related synthetic compounds on the rat superior cervical ganglion in situ, *Chem Pharm Bull* (Tokyo) 1974;22(6):1372-7.

Hsieh, C. et al. Anticonvulsant effect of Uncaria rhynchophylla (Miq) Jack. in rats with kainic acid-induced epileptic seizure, *Am J Chin Med* 1999;27(2): 257-64.

Jones, Kenneth. *Cat's Claw: Healing Vine of Peru*, Seattle, WA:Sylvan Press, 1995.

Kang, T. et al. Pteropodine and isopteropodine positively modulate the function of rat muscarinic M(1) and 5-HT(2) receptors expressed in Xenopus oocyte, *Eur J Pharmacol* 2002;444(1-2):39-45.

Kennedy, Ron. Lyme Disease and Cat's Claw. www.medical-library.net/sites/ _lyme_disease.htm. Accessed 8/23/2004.

Keplinger, K. et al. Oxindole alkaloids having properties stimulating the immunologic system, *United States Patent* 4,844,901, July 4, 1989.

———. Oxindole alkaloids having properties stimulating the immunologic system and preparation containing the same, *United States Patent* 4,940,725, July 10, 1990.

———. Oxindole alkaloids having properties stimulating the immunologic system and preparation containing the same, *United States Patent* 5,302,611, April 12, 1994. .

———. Process for the production of specific isomer mixtures from oxindole alkaloids, *United States Patent* 5,723,625, March 3, 1998.

———. Uncaria tomentosa (Willd.) DC—ethnomedical use and new pharmacological, toxicological, and botanical results, *J Ethnopharmacol* 1999;64(1):23-34.

Lamm, S. et al. Persistent response to pneumococcal vaccine in individuals supplemented with a novel water soluble extract of Uncaria tomentosa, C-Med-100, *Phytomedicine* 2001;8(4):267-74.

Lee, J. et al. Inhibition of phospholipase cgamma1 and cancer cell proliferation by triterpene esters from Uncaria rhynchophylla, *J Nat Prod* 2000;63(6):753-6.

Lemaire, I. et al. Stimulation of interleukin-1 and -6 production in alveolar macrophages by the neotropical liana, Uncaria tomentosa (una de gato), *J Ethnopharmacol* 1999;64(2): 109-15.

Liu, J. and Mori, A. Antioxidant and free radical scavenging activities of Gastrodia elata Bl. and Uncaria rhynchophylla (Miq.) Jacks, *Neuropharmacology* 1992;31(12): 1287-98.

Masumiya, H. et al. Effects of hirsutine and dihydrocorynantheine on the action potentials of sino-atrial node, atrium and ventricle, *Life Sci* 1999;65(22):2333-41.

Miller, M. et al. Dietary antioxidants protect gut epithelial cells from oxidant-induced apoptosis, *BMC Complement Altern Med* 2001;1(1):11.

Mimaki, Y. et al. Anti-convulsion effects of choto-san and chotoko (Uncariae Uncis cam Ramlus) in mice, and identification of the active principles, *Yakugaku Zasshi* 1997;117(12): 1011-21.

Mohamed, A. et al. Effects of Uncaria tomentosa total alkaloid and its components on experimental amnesia in mice: elucidation using the passive avoidance test, *J Pharm Pharmacol* 2000;52(120:1553-61.

Mok, J. et al. cardiovascular responses in the normotensive rat produced by intravenous infection of gambirine isolated from Uncaria callophylla Bl.ex Korth, *J Ethnopharmacol* 1992;36(3):219-23.

Muhammad, I. et al. Investigation of Una De gato I. 7-Deoxyloganic acid and (15)N NMR spectroscopic studies on pentacyclic oxindole alkaloids from Uncaria tomentosa, *Phytochemistry* 2001;57:781-5.

Mur, E. et al. Randomized double blind trial of an extract from the pentacyclic alkaloid-chemotype of uncaria tomentosa for the treatment of rheumatoid arthritis, *J Rheumatol* 2002;29(4):678-81.

Pengsuparp, T. et al. Pharmacological studies of geissoschizine methyl ether, isolated from Uncaria sinensis Oliv., in the central nervous system, *Eur J Pharmacol* 2001;425(3):211-18.

Pero, Ronald. Method of preparation and composition of a water soluble extract of the plant species Uncaria for enhancing immune, anti-inflammatory and anti-tumor processes of warm blooded animals, *United States Patent* 6,238,675, May 29, 2001.

———. Method of preparation and composition of a water soluble extract of the plant species Uncaria for enhancing immune, anti-inflammatory, anti-tumor and DNA repair processes of warm blooded animals, *United States Patent* 6,361,805, March 26, 2002.

Piscoya, J. et al. Efficacy and safety of freeze-dried cat's claw in osteoarthritis of the knee:mechanisms of action of the species Uncaria guianensis, *Inflamm Res* 2001;50(9):442-8.

Romanenko, A. et al. Traditional medicine in the prevention and treatment of Chernobyl radiation health consequences, www.manaxx.com/estudios-e2.htm.

Reinhard, K. Uncaria tomentosa (Willd.) D.C.:cat's claw, una de gato, or saventaro, *Journal of Alternative and Complementary Medicine* 1999;5(2): 143-51.

Riva, L. et al. The antiproliferative effects of Uncaria tomentosa extracts and fractions on the growth of breast cancer cell line, *Anticancer Res* 2001;21(4A):2457-61.

Rizzi, R. et al. Mutagenic and antimutagenic activities of Uncaria tomentosa and its extracts, *J Ethnopharmacol* 1993;38(1):63-77.

Rowan, Robert Jay. Chronic infections: some products and treatments that work, *Second Opinion* 2003;13(12):no page numbers available.

Sakakibara, I. et al. Effect on locomotion of indole alkaloids from the hooks of uncaria plants, *Phytomedicine* 1999;6(3):163-8.

Sandoval, M. et al. Anti-inflammatory and antioxidant activities of cat's claw (Uncaria tomentosa and Uncaria guianensis) are independent of their alkaloid content, *Phytomedicine* 2002;9(4):325-37.

———. Cat's claw inhibits TNFalpha production and scavenges free radicals: role in cytoprotection, *Free Radic Biol Med* 2000;29(1):71-8.

Sheng, Y. et al. DNA repair enhancement of aqueous extracts of Uncaria tomentosa in a human volunteer study, *Phytomedicine* 2001;8(4): 275-82.

———. Induction of apoptosis and inhibition of proliferation in human tumor cells treated with extracts of Uncaria tomentosa, *Anticancer Res* 1998;18(5A):3363-8.

———. Treatment of chemotherapy-induced leukopenia in a rat model with aqueous extract from Uncaria tomentosa, *Phytomedicine* 2000;7(2):137-43.

Shimada, Y. et al. Evaluation of the protective effects of alkaloids isolated from the hooks and stems of Uncaria sinensis on glutamate-induced neuronal death in cultured cerebellar granule cells from rats, *J Pharm Pharmacol* 1999;51(6):715-22.

———. Protective effect of phenolic compounds isolated from the hooks and stems of Uncaria sinensis on glutamate-induced neuronal death, *Am J Chin Med* 2001;29(10:173-80.

South, James. Samento:New remedy for an Ancient Enemy—Lyme Disease. www.samento.com.ec/sciencelib/sartic les/vrparticle.html. Accessed 10/7/2004.

Taylor, Leslie. The Cat's Claw TOA/POA Controversy (11-15-02). www.rain-tree.com/toa-poa-article.htm. Accessed 12/1/2004.

———. *Technical Data Report for Cat's Claw, "Una de gato," (Uncaria tomentosa)*, Austin, TX:Sage Press, 2002.

Tsuprykov, O. et al. Study of mechanism of immune effects, anti-viral and antineoplastic action of bioactive components of the preparation Manaxx, *International Conference on AIDS 2002 July 7-12*; 14 (abstract no. A10074).

Wagner, H. et al. The alkaloids of Uncaria tomentosa and their phagocytosis-stimulating actions, *Planta Med* 1985:419-23.

Walker, M and Walke, R. What Makes Lyme Disease Tick and How Samento Eliminates It. www.rense.com/general54/whatmakeslyme.htm. Accessed 8/23/2004.

Williams, James. Review of antiviral and immunomodulating properties of plants of the Peruvian rainforest with a particular emphasis on Una de Gato and Sangre de Grado, *Alternative medicine Review* 2001;6(6):567-579.

Winkler, C. et al. In vitro effects of two extracts and two pure alkaloid preparations of Uncaria tomentosa on peripheral blood mononuclear cells, *Planta Med* 2004;70(3):205-10.

Wurm M. et al. Pentacyclic oxindole alkaloids from Uncaria tomentosa induce endothelial cells to release a lymphocyte-proliferation-regulating factor. *Planta Med* 1998;64(8):701-4.

Yamahara, J. et al. Screening test for calcium antagonist in natural products. The active principles of Uncariae ramulus et uncus, *Nippon Yakurigaku Zasshi* 1987;90(3):133-40.

Zhu, M. et al. Application of radioligand receptor binding assays in the search for CNS active principles from Chinese medicinal plants, *J Ethnopharmacol* 1996;54(2-3):153-64.

HOMEOPATHY:

Allen, H.C. *Materia Medica of the Nosodes*, New Delhi, India:Jain Publishers, 1910 (1991).

Boericke, William. *Homeopathic Materia Medica*, Philadelphia, PA:Boericke and Taylor, 1927.

Castro, D. and Nogueira, G.G. Use of the nosode Meningococcinum as a preventative against meningitis, *Journal of the American Institute of Homeopathy* 1975;68:211-219.

Eisfelder, H.W. Poliomyelitis immunization—a final report. *Journal of the American Institute of Homeopathy* 1961; 144:166-67.

English, J.M. Pertussin 30—a preventative for Whooping Cough? A Pilot Study, *British Homeopathic Journal* 1987; 76:61-5.

Fine, Howard. Trigeminal neuralgia and palpitations from Lyme disease, *New England Journal of Homeopathy* 1998;7(1):59-62.

Gardner, Cindee. Treating Lyme disease naturally. www.hpathy.com/papersnew. Accessed 5/8/2004.

Griggs, W. Thirty years of clinical research and confirmation of the intestinal nosode dysentery co. *J Am Inst Homeopath* 1966;59(7):238-40.

Guess, George. A subacute case of Lyme disease, *New England Journal of Homeopathy* 1998;7(1):57-8.

Jonas, W. Do homeopathic nosodes protect against infection? An experimental test. *Altern Ther Health Med* 1999;5(5):36-40.

Levy, Jeff. A small remedy in (alleged) Lyme disease in a dog, *New England Journal of Homeopathy* 1998;7(1): 62-5.

Malerba, Larry. A case of Lyme related neuropathy, *New England Journal of Homeopathy* 1998;7(1):41-6.

————. Ticked off by a tick, *New England Journal of Homeopathy* 1998; 7(1):47-52.

Neustaedter, Randall. *The Vaccine Guide*, Berkeley, CA:North Atlantic Books, 2002.

Rothenberg, Amy. If you hear hoofbeats, don't think zebras—a case of chronic Lyme disease, *New England Journal of Homeopathy* 2000; 9(2):73-8.

Rotundo, Beth. Lyme with the desire to kill, *New England Journal of Homeopathy* 1998;7(1):53-6.

Tobin, Stephen. Lyme disease and homeopathy. www.cassia.org/ledum.htm. Accessed 5/29/2004.

Tyler, M.L. *Homeopathic Drug Pictures*, Third Edition, Essex, England: C.W.Daniel Company, 1952.

Ullman, Dana. *Homeopathic Medicine for Children and Infants*, NY:Tarcher/Perigee, 1992.

Whitmont, Ronald. Homeopathy and Lyme disease. www.homeopathicmd.com/articles_3.html. Accessed 10/12/2004.

Yasgur, Jay. *Yasgur's Homeopathic Dictionary*, Fourth edition, Greenville, PA:Van Hoy Publishers, 1998.

INDEX